CHAPTER		PAGE
I	INTRODUCTORY	1
II	COLETTE MAKES SOUP	4
III	COLETTE COOKS EGGS	18
IV	FRENCH RAGOUTS AND STEWS	32
V	COLETTE COOKS BIRDS AND BEASTS	44
VI	COLETTE AND THE LEFT-OVERS	63
VII	COLETTE AND THE CHAFING DISH	74
VIII	COLETTE COOKS FISH	84
IX	OUT OF THE FRYING PAN	94
X	COLETTE COOKS VEGETABLES	109
XI	COLETTE MAKES SAUCES	127
XII	COLETTE MAKES CANDIED FRUITS AND SWEETS	138
XIII	COLETTE MAKES CAKES AND BISCUITS	151
XIV	COLETTE COOKS FRUIT	168
XV	COLETTE MAKES CREAMS AND SWEET DISHES	181

Colette's Best Recipes

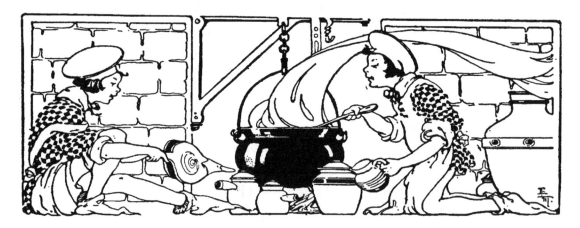

CHAPTER I

INTRODUCTORY

"COLETTE, were you ever anything but a cook?"

"Yes, once. In my first place, I was cowherd. I was eight years and three months old, and my mother had put me to service on a farm, because there were too many mouths to fill at home. But, one day, the mistress of that farm had a baby — suddenly, you understand — and there was no one to make the soup for the man. So they fetched me in from the long pasture, and I did it. I liked it better than herding — so much better that I was glad when she died — that unfortunate one! — and the sudden baby, too, and left me to make the soup always. I did not mean to think wickedly, you understand well. But I was young and without education — and she had given me a slap or two, now and then — and I loved to make the soup. I have made it ever since."

"And that was — *how* long ago?"

"Fifty-one years in August."

Colette's Best Recipes

"Fifty-one years of cooking! And yet you do not seem tired of it!"

"I am not. For, look you, in the cooking there is always something new to learn, something new to try. There are as many different ways of cooking a chicken as he has feathers on his back. And then times change, and seasons change, and to-day you are rich and to-morrow you are poor, and the cooking must fit itself to all that comes. Oh, no! It is not possible that a woman, who knows a little about cooking and interests herself in it, should find it dull. It is only the Shiftless Ones — those who muddle along anyhow — who find it wearisome. I pity them! From my heart I pity them! Fancy doing *bad* cooking! How it must lie on the conscience, not to speak of the stomach!"

"Perhaps they know no better—" I begin, taking up arms to defend a world full of Shiftless Ones. But Colette will accept no weak excuses.

"Perhaps they did not know better *up till now*. Let us suppose so in charity. But now I have told them better. I have told them how to cook as a Christian — as a Frenchwoman — should. *You* know that I have told them, for you wrote it down yourself on that writing machine of yours, all the afternoons of last summer, when I had made the kitchen clean, and cleared the table for you. They have nothing to do but read the book, and then they will know all that I have learned about cooking in fifty-one years."

As a matter of fact, you *won't* — not half or a quarter of it. No single book could be made to contain all the floods of information that Colette poured out on me during those summer afternoons. But some of it is here, anyway, — as many recipes as I could squeeze in, and a certain amount of general instruction.

Do you think you could find time to read right through

Introductory

the book, please? It is not a work of reference; it is a gossip in a kitchen. If you only turn up in the index the recipe you want, and read just that, the chances are great that your dish will fail for lack of a little hint or warning which comes somewhere else in the chapter. And we should hate to have you spoil anything, Colette and I.

But I don't believe you will. For this book deals only with the French *cuisine de famille;* and that — like most other very good things and very good folks — is simplicity itself.

CHAPTER II

COLETTE MAKES SOUP

SO, you see, Colette's career began with the soup. Many things do, in France, — the two chief meals of every day, for instance, in every family; and some things end with it also, as, in many working-class homes, there is nothing else for dinner and supper except just the soup, and a big hunk of bread to dip in it. And, on that, the boys and girls manage to grow up as strong and active and wiry as you please. For there is no more valuable article of food than well-made soup.

Mind, it must be well made. A soup square, melted down in a little hot water or a highly seasoned mess out of a tin have no food value at all, or next to none. Besides, they are very costly, and quite needlessly so: real, home-made soup should cost next to nothing, as all the odds and ends in the house can be used up for it.

Roughly speaking, soups can be divided into three classes: PURÉES, or soups that have been rubbed through a sieve or a colander; BREAD SOUPS (specially French in nature); CLEAR SOUPS.

Let me try to give you a notion of each in turn. You should always remember that, in the first two categories the word "stock" means either meat boilings or vegetable water. Special stock made from bones is quite unnecessary.

Colette Makes Soup

Remember also, please, that the time given for cooking is the *shortest possible one*. Soups can nearly always be cooked, with advantage, for an almost unlimited length of time. All those that do not contain either eggs or whole pieces of bread or toast can be warmed up, and will improve, rather than otherwise, in the process.

BREAD SOUPS

PANADE is the first soup that a French baby gets. In schools over here, they give it to the children for breakfast, in place of any other cereal. It can also be served at dinner, though only " in the family."

Allow a good half slice of bread for each person. The more crusts you can use, the nicer will be the *panade*. Put it into a big pot with plenty of water, and boil steadily, but not too fast, for one hour. Don't stir! If you do, the bread will sink to the bottom and burn.

Drain out the bread. Put it through a sieve or colander. If you want plain Panade à l'Eau, such as school children get, thin it out with its water to the consistency of a soup, season it with salt and a very little sugar, and reheat it, *stirring all the while*. Just before it is done add a lump of butter, more or less generous, according to your resources.

PANADE AU LAIT. After the bread has gone through the sieve, thin it out with boiling milk. Add sugar, and just a wee pinch of salt, with butter to taste. This is the staple food of French babies.

PANADE À LA REINE. Make it just like Panade au Lait. But, after it has boiled up the second time, draw the pan off the fire and beat in the yolks of one or two eggs. Return the pan and stir constantly while the eggs thicken, but do not let the soup boil again. This is very often served to invalids, or to children when they need a treat.

Colette's Best Recipes

PANADE À L'OIGNON (ONION POTAGE). Allow one small onion for each person. Boil them with the bread, and put them through the sieve with it. Thin out the soup either with its own water, or with meat boilings. This is excellent for colds, and for all skin troubles. Season well with salt and pepper, but keep just a wee grain of sugar too; it helps the taste of the onion.

PANADE AUX LÉGUMES (VEGETABLE POTAGE). When you have cold vegetables left, mix them into the hot bread as you drain it out of the pan, and put all through the sieve together. Thin out the mixture with vegetable water. This is a good family soup.

SOUPE À L'OSEILLE BLANCHIE (WHITE SORREL SOUP). Take a big double handful of tender young sorrel, which has been washed and picked over. Put it in the soup pan with a lump of butter the size of an egg, and stir over the fire till the leaves soften. Add one and a half quarts of water or stock. Let the whole thing boil five minutes. Now cut about six largish and very thin slices of bread. Throw them into the pan, draw it aside, cover it, and let it simmer gently for quarter of an hour. Now beat up the yolks of two eggs with salt, pepper, and a little of the warm soup. Stir them in just at the moment of service. Have ready the whites, beaten to a stiff froth with a little salt. If you use a soup tureen, dab the whole big lump of white into it. If you serve in plates, put a white tuft on each plate.

This soup is "very foreign looking" and never fails to attract comment from those who have not lived in France.

Soupe à la Bretonne (Brittany Soup)

3 large onions   A handful of sorrel or spinach
2 small carrots   A piece of butter the size of an egg
2 small turnips   1 quart stock or water
          Slices — or rather shavings — of stale bread

Colette Makes Soup

Peel the vegetables and cut them into very small dice. The green stuff should be washed and cut into fine strips. Put them into the soup pan with the butter, and let them get well warmed through. Then add the liquid and boil steadily for two hours. Add salt and pepper to taste.

Now take a stale loaf — or, better still, a big crusty roll — and cut off from it the thinnest possible shavings. They should not be slices, but real shavings, curled and ragged. Put at least six, and more if you like, of these shavings into each plate. Pour in boiling soup, taking care that you give a fair share of vegetables with each serving. Cover the plates, and stand them beside the fire, or in a cool oven, for five minutes, so that the bread may soak: then add as much more soup as each plate will hold, and serve.

JULIENNE AU PAIN (JULIENNE, WITH BREAD) is very much the same kind of thing, except that you must take all the root vegetables you can lay hands on in equal amounts, and no green stuff at all, unless you happen to have some green peas. Cut all the vegetables small. Be generous with the butter in which you warm them. Cook just as above, but, when it comes to a question of the bread, cut neat thin slices, just large enough to fit tidily into your soup plates, and toast them very brown indeed.

SOUPE MOUSSELINE. Melt three ounces of butter in the soup pan. Add a handful of spinach or sorrel, carefully washed, picked, and cut into fine strips. When the green begins to change color, add one quart of water and half a pound of the white of bread. Salt and pepper the soup to taste, and let it simmer one hour.

Now beat up the yolks of two eggs with one pint of very hot milk. Stir in the whites, beaten to the firmest possible froth. Pour all into the soup tureen — which should be

Colette's Best Recipes

well heated first — and then add the soup, little by little, beating all the while. Serve at once.

This is rather an old-fashioned soup, which still remains in favor, and might quite well appear on a dinner menu.

CROÛTE AU POT (CRUST IN THE POT) is another well-known national soup. It can only be made with meat boilings, — not with vegetable water.

Toast two thin slices of bread and put them in the soup pan with the fatty part from the top of the boiling meat pot. At first there should be enough liquid to cover them. But, as they boil, the liquor will evaporate, leaving them to stick to the bottom of the pot. When they are well stuck, take them off carefully with a knife, put them in the soup tureen, and pour over them the meat boilings, nicely seasoned.

If you can use crusts of bread, rather than slices with white in them, so much the better.

Now let us have a few purées.

Their name is legion, for every kind of vegetable is capable of being boiled and then put through a sieve: and the more different kinds you mix together, the more various and interesting will your purées be. Here are a few examples.

SOUPE DE DIVERS LÉGUMES (MIXED VEGETABLE SOUP). Add together all the vegetable waters and meat boilings that you have, up to two quarts. Put all on to boil. When it boils, add whatever vegetables may be in season, — carrots, turnips, onions, parsnips, peas, celery, and either old potatoes or haricot beans, to thicken the entire affair. You must never have less than three vegetables, of which one must be onions and one the thickening. When all are soft, put all through a colander with big holes. Reheat it, stirring all the while. Add salt, pepper, and the largest lump of butter or good dripping that you can spare.

Colette Makes Soup

This soup keeps several days, reheats perfectly, and is capable of variation by the addition of any vegetables you happen to have, provided that they are already cooked.

SOUPE D'HARICOTS (HARICOT BEAN SOUP). Wash and soak one pound of haricot beans. Put them on to boil with four large peeled potatoes, four large peeled onions, and two quarts of water or stock. Boil till the beans are perfectly tender. Then put the whole thing through a sieve. It will be quite thick, and you should not thin it out. Reheat it, stirring carefully. Just before serving, add salt and pepper to taste, and the biggest lump of butter you can spare.

This is a very nourishing soup, — just what you want for the family dinner on cold-meat days.

SOUPE DE LENTILLES OU DE POIS (PEA OR LENTIL SOUP). This is very similar. Use dried peas, either green or yellow, or dried lentils. Measure them, soak them overnight, and add four times as much of water as you have of vegetables. Add also one onion and one large carrot to each pint of liquid. Cook just as above, adding a tiny wee pinch of sugar, as well as the salt and pepper, just before serving, if the soup has been made with water or vegetable stock. If it has been made with meat boilings, you will find just a very small dash of made mustard nicer than the sugar.

SOUPE AUX POMMES DE TERRE (POTATO SOUP). There are almost an unlimited number of flavorings for potato soup, — onion, celery, salsify, mixed herbs being the favorites. Whichever you choose, it should be cooked in with the soup.

Allow five large potatoes to one quart stock or water. Peel them, boil them in the stock till they are soft, and put them through a fine sieve. Reheat the whole affair, adding a generous lump of butter. At the moment of service, stir in one fourth the amount of milk — or, better still, of cream

— heated, but not boiling, that you used of stock. Unless you are very sure of the freshness of your cream mix it first with a little boiling soup in a basin: it would be such a shame if you were to put it straight into the whole quantity, and then have to stand and watch it turn!

SOUPE AUX CHOUX (CABBAGE SOUP) is a very great specialty of Colette's, and I think I will put it in here, though it is not exactly a purée. There are several different kinds.

1. Put on a big pot holding at least two quarts of water, and throw into it

4 carrots, cut into long thin strips
6 onions, roughly chopped
1 cupful haricot beans, soaked
4 large potatoes, peeled
A cupful of green peas, if you have any
A bunch of mixed herbs
A couple of cloves, stuck into a little onion, which is there especially for them
A good-sized cabbage, with the stalks and the outer leaves removed, and the rest cut into rough pieces
Salt and pepper

Cover the pot and boil hard for three hours. Then add a piece of butter or good dripping, the size of two eggs. Boil for half an hour more. Fish out the potatoes, if they are not already in pulp, and smash them roughly. Finish off the soup by throwing in little dice of crust, which should just have time to soak before it is served.

This is a real good farmhouse soup, — the sort that you almost live on when you spend a holiday in the country. If you can make it of the water in which a ham, or a large piece of bacon, has been boiled, it is delicious.

2. SOUPE AUX CHOUX ET AU FROMAGE (CABBAGE AND CHEESE SOUP). This cannot be made except in a soup tureen.

Colette Makes Soup

Put at the bottom of the tureen a layer of small, thin pieces of bread. On them sprinkle a layer of grated Parmesan cheese. Then more bread. Then more cheese. Then a final layer of bread. Having made a Soupe aux Choux, as above, ladle a little of the liquid into the tureen, — enough to soak the bread very well. Cover the tureen, and stand it at the side of the fire for three quarters of an hour, so that the bread may soak. Then pour in the rest of the soup and serve.

This, according to Colette, is "a much more presentable soup", and worth careful making. Cut the vegetables into wee dice, or even stamp them out with a tiny cutter: but leave the pieces of cabbage rather big, or you will take away all the character of the dish.

3. SOUPE AUX CHOUX À LA VIANDE (CABBAGE AND MEAT SOUP). When you have had a roast, either of beef or mutton, which was rather underdone, leave a little of the meat clinging to the bone, saw the bone at three or four places, and boil it in the Soupe aux Choux. You need not, in this case, use any butter at all. Colette often adds a good handful of rice when she uses a bone: in this case, no bread is needed.

Last of all come the clear soups, which are, as a rule, considered finer and better than the thick ones. There is a sort of "halfway house" of a soup, which gets served continually in every French family, and is a triumph of economy, both in money and effort. It is called POT-AU-FEU (POT-ON-THE-FIRE), and it is made by the very simple expedient of taking a nice piece of boiling beef and cooking it in a big pot, with all the vegetables you have handy. At the end of five to seven hours of cooking, fish out the beef — which will be perfectly tender — slice it, and serve it hot, covered with any of the meat sauces which you will find in Chapter XI. Or an even simpler — and more really French — way of doing things is just to slice the beef, arrange the slices at the middle of a dish, fish out of the pot enough vegetables to make a pretty border, and pour a little of the pot liquor over all. Serve the soup first, with bread broken into it, and you have the staple dinner of the French middle-class household, comparable to a meal of roast mutton and bread pudding in England.

Colette wants you to know that there is a rule of procedure in the making of *Pot-au-feu*, and it is this:

Put the beef into cold water and bring it to a boil.

Skim it carefully.

Add the vegetables, peeled and cut into moderate pieces, but not too small. Carrots, for instance, may be split into four lengthwise bits, and an ordinary cabbage cut into six pieces. But, as the pot must boil for so long, there is no need to hurry the cooking of the vegetables by cutting them smaller.

Let it boil up and skim it once more.

Add salt. Cover the pot. Keep it boiling at any rate you like. If you don't want to use the meat that day, let it soak in the soup all night, and just warm them up together next morning.

A piece of beef weighing five pounds is enough to make a gallon of good *Pot-au-feu*.

BOUILLON, which is the foundation of most clear soups, can be made with meat or bones of any kind. Colette seldom buys soup meat; indeed, she would think it almost a crime to do so. But, as we live in a country where butchers bone their meat as a matter of course — except the large joints of beef and mutton — each piece that comes into the house brings its little pile of detached bones for the soup pot.

The best of all, without doubt, are veal bones, which

Colette Makes Soup

make a delicious, jelly-like soup. Beef and mutton bones are a little tasteless, but can be improved by being chopped here and there, so that the marrow may come out. Game and chicken bones and leavings are excellent, and Colette always says that the fore quarters of a rabbit do better work in the soup pot than on the dish. (There is little to eat on them, you know, but they give an excellent flavor.) You can mix several different kinds of meat with advantage, and I need hardly remind you, I think, that the water in which a tongue, ham, or bit of bacon has been boiled is a perfect treasure for the soup pot. When people are coming to dinner, Colette nearly always puts a pair of pig's feet into the bouillon, for there is nothing that gives a more delicious flavor. And I like them very much to eat, cold, next day, with a little mayonnaise dressing.

First and last, you should have one pound of bones or bits of meat to each two pints of water, if you want to get a real, good, strong bouillon. If you want it to keep well, use no vegetables, as they tend to make it turn, — nothing but the meat, the water, and a little salt.

Boil, with the lid on the pan, for at least five hours, and as many more as you can manage. Let the bouillon get cold. Skim it most carefully and save the skimmings for frying. There's nothing more tasty than sauté potatoes made with the skimmings of a well-seasoned bouillon.

Strain out as much as you want to use at a time, keeping the big pot of soup in a cool place, and boiling it up every two days in warm weather, and every three days in cold, if it lasts that long. It may be used in any of the following ways:

VERMICELLE AU GRAS. Salt and pepper the bouillon to taste, color it with a little browning, make it boil up fast, and break in vermicelli. Stir till it boils again. Cook fifteen minutes, and serve.

Colette's Best Recipes

POTAGE OF ITALIAN PASTE. Make it exactly like the Vermicelle soup. When it is served, have a plate of grated Parmesan added, so that each person may help himself.

POTAGE AU MACARONI, TAPIOCA, etc., are all made just the same. Large macaroni takes thirty-five minutes to cook in the soup, and tapioca more or less time, according to size: but, when it is quite clear, you may know that it is done.

POTAGE AUX CROÛTONS FRITES. Serve a perfectly plain bouillon, and hand wee stars of fried bread with it; or, better still, use

CHOUX PUFFS. Put into a pan one fourth pint of water, two and one half ounces of flour, and one ounce of butter. Let them boil. Then draw the pan aside and stir in two and one half ounces of flour. Beat smooth with a wooden spoon. Return the pan to the fire and stir again till the paste just begins to bubble. Then draw the pan away once more and beat in an egg. When the egg is most thoroughly mixed, let the paste stand to get cold. Then heat your pan of deep fat to smoking point, take up the weest possible little bits of paste, and drop them in. They puff up enormously, and turn a bright biscuit brown at once. Drain them, store them in a tin, and just reheat them a little in the oven before serving, to make them crisp. Hand them with clear soup. They look ever so nice and taste delicious. The quantities that I have given you make a big tin full, — enough to last quite a while.

When you are making pastry, save up all the odds and ends, roll them into long thin strips, and, holding a strip over a pan of frying fat, heated to smoking point, snip off the end in wee bits, which fall down into the pan. They puff and swim up to the top almost at once, and are deliciously crisp and nice with the bouillon.

Colette Makes Soup

JULIENNE. You must use for this a good mixture of root vegetables — at least four different kinds — and, if possible, green peas with them. The whole art of preparing the Julienne lies in the cutting up of the various roots in very wee bits, none of them larger than a pea. When all are done, put them into the soup pan with one ounce butter for each pint of vegetables, and cook gently till the vegetables begin to soften. Then add a quart of good bouillon — or more, if you like — for each pint of vegetables: boil three quarters of an hour: serve with little snips of fried bread.

The bouillon may be colored or left plain, according to taste. It should be well seasoned with pepper and salt.

POTAGE PRINTANIÈRE (SPRING SOUP). This is pretty much the same kind of thing, except that asparagus points, green peas, and wee spring onions are essential to it. (You probably won't get anything much else to put with them at that season of the year.) Add a little white sugar to the soup, tasting carefully after each pinch that you stir in.

POTAGE AU MELON (MELON SOUP). This is perfectly delicious. Peel and seed a small melon, and cut the fruit into neat, small cubes, not more than one and one half inches in size. Boil them till tender in plain water. Drain them.

Slice one large onion into the soup pan and fry it in a heaped tablespoonful of butter. Pour on to it one quart of boiling bouillon, add the melon, season to taste with salt and pepper. Simmer for five minutes before serving.

BOUILLON À LA MINUTE (HASTY SOUP). Take one fourth pint of gravy from the roast, — beef, mutton, or veal. Skim it most carefully, taking away every possible drop of dripping. Add it to one pint of boiling vegetable water or plain water. Serve with choux puffs or fried bread. Very good indeed.

CONSOMMÉ is not much used except in illness or for very grand occasions. But you may like to know how to make it, all the same.

4 pints water
2 lbs. lean beef
An old bird of any kind — game or hen — or the fore quarters of a rabbit or hare
2 each of carrots, onions, and parsnips
A bunch of sweet herbs
2 cloves, stuck into one of the onions

Boil for eight hours. Let it cool and skim carefully. This makes a really splendid consommé. The meat can be used a second time in the family soup pot, though I do not suppose there will be so very much richness left in it.

"For all the other clear soups," says Colette, "let folks just take notice, when they go out to dinner, of what they are eating, and they will get no end of ideas. Clear soup is always clear soup: and, when you find that it has been improved by the addition of this little thing, or that little thing, — well, all you have to do is to notice just what it may be, and put it in your own pot next time. What could be easier?"

If you want to make good soup always:

1. Add the seasoning at the very end, unless the recipe tells you something different. There are certain seasonings — cloves, for instance — which must be cooked in the soup. But salt and pepper, which are the most ordinary seasonings, should generally be added at the last moment, with a careful stir-up and an attentive tasting between each pinch.

2. If your soup is too salty, or rather dull in taste, add

Colette Makes Soup

a very little rough brown sugar. It is often a great help in bringing out other flavors.

3. Remember that bread thickenings and pressed purées must hardly ever be stirred at the first boiling while the ingredients are whole: but when they are reheated, after being put through the sieve, they must be stirred continually and kept on a very moderate heat, for they will burn if you give them the smallest chance.

4. If soup burns, never stir or jolt it, but take the pan off the fire at once, holding it very steady, and gently pour the contents into a clean vessel. As soon as you see that burnt bits are beginning to pour out, stop. Throw the rest away. Never, on any account, scrape the pan or help the soup out with a spoon. Carry the clean vessel out into the fresh air and there taste the soup. (You cannot do a fair tasting in the kitchen, where your nose and mouth will be full of tainted air.) If the scorched taste is very slight, reheat the soup, adding to it a good bunch of fresh mint, and it will be eatable, though I do not promise that it will be good. But if the scorched taste is strong, don't waste time and trouble on it. Throw it right away, for if you serve scorched soup even once, it is so nasty that you run the risk of disgusting your folks forever with this useful dish.

5. If you are making soup with cold vegetables, which is sometimes a very handy thing to do, don't try to boil them up in the soup pot, or they will surely sink to the bottom and scorch. Boil the water or bouillon or whatever it is, and pour it on them, just let them warm and soften a little, and then put them through a sieve and reheat them like a fresh purée.

CHAPTER III

COLETTE COOKS EGGS

WHEN the Story-teller said that she wanted to come and stay, I was ever so pleased. For a long while I had liked and admired her at a respectful distance; and the thought of having her under my own roof and all to myself was enchanting. But there was just one thorn in my rose-leaf bed. The Story-teller is a food faddist of a most pronounced type; and what was Colette going to say about that?

I mentioned gently that a lady was coming to stay on Saturday. Colette looked pleased. She likes visitors.

"I will kill the little pig — the one with a black spot near his tail," said she.

"But that's just the trouble," I explained; "this lady eats no meat."

"The fish merchant passes only on Thursdays," said Colette hastily. (She detests fish, and cooks it worse than anything else.)

"She doesn't eat fish either. She lives entirely on eggs."

Colette screwed up her brown old face into the most severe of wrinkles. "Is she a *fin bec?*" demanded she.

I hesitated. But truth and a cold in the head must come out, sooner or later, so — "Well — perhaps — just a little," I admitted. And I waited, shaking in my shoes.

The wrinkles deepened, wavered, broke, and the whole

Colette Cooks Eggs

face beamed in a broad grin of pure delight. "Ah! *Merci, mon Dieu!*" cried Colette devoutly. "At last I shall have in the house somebody who will really eat and enjoy eggs as they ought to be cooked! Does she stay long, this lady?"

"Fifteen days."

"And she will eat eggs twice a day! *Encore un grand merci, mon Dieu!*" She was quite carried away over it.

The Story-teller had n't been in the house an hour before she and Colette had fallen on each other's necks, and the result was that Colette's egg-cooking became not only an artistic triumph, but a work of love. Really, she did some remarkably good things — and quite out of the way, many of them. I will try to tell you about them.

The first evening, there was a sort of creamy dish, with green peas in it, and wee stars of fried bread to decorate the edge. "ŒUFS AUX PETITS POIS," murmured the Story-teller. "I ate it often in Paris, but it was not as good as this — the peas were less completely mixed into the eggs. I think they cooked the eggs first, and put the peas in afterwards, and —"

"Ah! But that is wrong!" cried Colette, quite forgetting that she must not talk when she waits at table. "Listen! This is how I do it:

"I fry my little stars of bread and keep them very hot in the oven till they are wanted. I take one pint of tender little peas, wash them in cold water, drain them well, and toss them in as much flour as they can pick up. In my casserole, I melt a big tablespoonful of butter, and toss the peas in it till they are well buttered all over. Then I add one half pint of water, one half teaspoonful of salt, one big lump of sugar, and one little onion, peeled."

"Or one bay leaf," suggested the Story-teller.

"If you choose. Or, again, one may rub the sugar on a cut bead of garlic. All are good. Bring the pan to the boil, cover it, let it simmer till the peas are quite tender.

"Now beat up four eggs as if for an omelette. Move your pan to a hot place on the fire. Pour in the eggs and stir briskly with a little wooden spoon till they *just* take. Whisk the pan off the fire at once, pour the contents into a hot dish, decorate with the fried bread, and serve without losing a second.

"The important thing is that the eggs must not be allowed to harden into lumps, as badly cooked scrambled eggs do, for example. There is just one moment at which, mingling with the sauce from the peas, they make a thick, smooth cream. And that moment is the one in which you must whisk your pan off the fire. Wateriness means that they are done too little, and lumpiness that they are done too much. Only creaminess is perfection."

If new peas are not to be had, one can very nicely use those that are canned. Drain them and toss them in flour as directed above. In a double boiler melt a generous tablespoonful of butter, and add a small onion, grated; then put in the peas and stir until the butter is sizzling. Then add the water, salt, and a lump (or teaspoonful) of sugar and proceed in exactly the same way as with fresh peas.

Next day at lunch there was a little copper saucepan standing before the Story-teller's place. It was a pretty little saucepan, beautifully cleaned and twinkling invitingly; still, one does not, as a rule, put pans on the table, and I began to murmur an excuse.

"It's all right!" she assured me. "That's a FONDU AU FROMAGE, and it always must be served in the thing in which it is cooked, in order to be hot enough. Some people

Colette Cooks Eggs

use a copper or fireproof china dish, but I like the saucepan best, myself — more unusual."

A FONDU AU FROMAGE is quite easy to make. Break into your little pan four very fresh eggs. Add a big pinch of pepper, a small pinch of salt, and a big pinch of sugar, and beat the whole thing with a wooden spoon till the eggs froth well. Then add two ounces of fresh butter and four ounces of grated cheese — Cheddar or Gruyère — set the pan on a very gentle heat, and stir continually with a wooden spoon till the mixture thickens into a smooth cream.

Again, this mustn't be allowed to go into lumps, like an omelette or scrambled eggs. As soon as it clings to the spoon and coats it, it is done. Serve it in the pan and give something crisp and crackling to eat with it; potato ribbons, piping hot, sprinkled well with salt, and piled up on a folded napkin, are the ideal.

ŒUFS AU FROMAGE (CHEESE EGGS). Colette considers this one of the most nourishing of all her egg dishes, — quite substantial enough to be the chief course of a meal. She always serves purée of potatoes with it, as the dish itself is rather rich, and can well carry off a simple vegetable, such as mashed potatoes.

Allow two eggs for each person; more if you like, of course, but two at least. Get your pan of deep frying fat on the fire, and heat it till it comes to boiling point, which it does just a few seconds before it stops bubbling and gives off a thin blue smoke. Then drop the eggs in, one at a time, and poach them in the fat, just as you are accustomed to do in water. They cook much faster in the fat, and you should be ready to take them out as soon as they are set. If you allow them to harden, the charm of the dish will be lost. Have ready a fireproof dish in which you have melted one half teaspoonful of the best fresh butter, and one tablespoonful of grated cheese for each egg. The dish should stand in the oven while you are preparing the eggs, and you should stir the contents now and then, so that the cheese may melt nicely without getting browned at all. Arrange the eggs neatly in the prepared dish, spoon just a little of the butter over them, sprinkle them daintily with salt and pepper, and serve the whole thing piping hot. Take care to drain the eggs when you fish them out of the fat.

If you cannot eat rich things, poach the eggs in water. But the dish becomes more ordinary at once, though still nice.

ŒUFS À L'ARDENNAISE. "Almost as uncommon as it is delicious," sighed the Story-teller, lovingly regarding the snowy mountains of whipped white, with golden yolks tucked away amongst them. " Why don't folks do it more often, I wonder? It is quite easy."

Take a rather deep fireproof dish and butter it. Whip up the whites of four or five eggs to a froth so stiff that the fork will stand in it, seasoning them with pepper, salt, a tiny pinch of mixed sweet herbs, just as if for an omelette. Pile the whipped whites roughly in the dish and trickle over them one tablespoonful of good cream for each egg. Slip in the yolks wherever they fit best, and set the whole thing in a brisk oven till the yolks are *just* set. The white really ought not to brown, although, now and then, one can't keep it from coloring a little on the peaks. Serve immediately in the dish in which it is cooked.

"What a pity that Madame can take no meat!" sighed Colette regretfully. "It hinders me from making her an OMELETTE AUX CROÛTONS, which is the best of all omelettes."

"Oh, but I don't go as far as that!" the Story-teller assured her hastily. "It is not that I have made a vow

Colette Cooks Eggs

against meat, my good Colette. It is simply that slices of beef and mutton do not agree with me. But an Omelette aux Croûtons made with a little gravy of veal or chicken — why, that is all that there is of the most delicious, is it not?"

It was. And not quite like any other omelette that I have ever tasted.

Take a good round of bread about one fourth inch thick, remove the crusts, and cut the white into little squares, fry the squares in a very little butter, till they are just colored. Now put into a pan a very small drop of good gravy — just enough to cover the bottom to the depth of about one inch — put in your fried bread, let them drink up all they can, and then add more if necessary, so that the pan is just *not* dry. Let it stand at the side of the fire and simmer gently till the bread is quite tender, adding a few drops more of gravy if they are wanted, but remembering that, in the end, the pan *must boil dry*. Beat it up with a fork, add salt and pepper to taste — if the gravy was not already sufficiently seasoned — and then beat in four eggs, one at a time. Have ready a little butter melted in an omelette pan, pour in the mixture, and cook exactly like an ordinary omelette, taking care that it does not stick, which it will be rather inclined to do on account of the bread in it.

ŒUFS MOLLETS AUX FINES HERBES (HERB EGGS). Colette gave us Œufs Mollets several times. In France, they are served very frequently — all kinds of different sauces being put with them, — tomato, cream sauce, thickened gravies, etc. They are quite easy to do, and many people find them far more digestible than hard-boiled eggs.

Bring a pan of water to the boil, drop in your eggs, and let them boil fast for five minutes. Fish them out and drop them straight into the coldest water you can get. Let them stop in the cold water just one minute. Then take them out and peel them immediately. They are not quite easy to do at first, as the shells rather tend to stick to the whites; but a little practice will give you the trick of it. Eggs cooked in this way are well set and yet tender to the touch, and with the full taste, which is lost when they are boiled hard. Have your sauce ready and pour it over them at once, before they have time to get cold.

Supposing that you want to do them *aux fines herbes*, you must make the characteristic and delicious sauce.

Put into a small saucepan one teaspoonful chopped parsley, one teaspoonful grated onion or shallot, one leaf of mint and a tiny leaf of laurel, the juice of a large sweet-orange, three tablespoonfuls water, and a large tablespoonful of butter, rolled in as much flour as it can pick up. Let all boil gently for one fourth hour, stirring often, and adding a little more water if the sauce gets too thick. Strain it. Add salt and pepper to taste. Put the eggs into an *au gratin* dish, pour the sauce over them, sprinkle with fine crumbs of fried bread, and just slip the dish into the oven for long enough to heat it all up thoroughly, but not long enough either to dry the sauce or harden the eggs.

"In Italy, they leave out the butter, laurel, mint, and onion, and, instead, they use oil and garlic and just about half of a leaf of sage," said the Story-teller. "I don't know that their dish is better than yours, my Colette — no, that I do not say — but you might try it, one time, by way of a change."

ŒUFS À L'AIL (GARLIC EGGS). "You cannot meet any one after you have eaten it — you will smell too strongly of garlic," Colette warned us.

"I do not want to meet any one who is narrow-minded

Colette Cooks Eggs

enough to object to garlic," the Story-teller reassured her regarding the tempting looking salad lovingly. "How did you make it, Colette?"

Cook six beads of garlic in just enough water to cover them for ten minutes. Then drain them and pound them in a mortar with two anchovies and six capers. When they are crushed to a smooth paste stir in three tablespoonfuls of olive oil, one and one half tablespoonfuls of vinegar, and pepper and salt to taste.

Cut four hard-boiled eggs in quarters, pile them up at the middle of a rather flat salad dish, pour the dressing over them, and make a light border of cress or small salad.

"Could you do it with shallots instead of garlic?" asked the Story-teller.

"Why, yes. It is weak, you know — poor — a sort of second-best. But those who have not been brought up on garlic — who have not their palates formed to it — might like the shallots better. If you use shallots, put in just a tiny dab of made mustard. It helps them — brings out the taste — makes them more interesting."

ŒUFS MIMOSA was the prettiest and most tempting thing Colette had ever done, I thought, though the two egg epicures shook their heads sadly at my lack of taste, and said it was "ordinary."

Boil four eggs hard, and drop them into cold water as soon as they are done, won't you, to keep the yolks from turning green outside? Cut them in halves lengthwise. Remove the yolks. Make a nice stiff mayonnaise with the yolk of a very fresh egg, and pile it in the spaces left in the whites. At the center of a flat dish make a small round pile of finely chopped small salad, tossed in just a drop or two of oil and vinegar. Put the prepared whites all round, radiating outwards from the pile, like the petals of a flower. Hold a fine sieve over the dish, and rub the hard-boiled yolks through it, so that they fall in fine golden rain. Cool it well before serving.

GÂTEAU DORÉ (GOLDEN CAKE). It's not a cake at all, but a sort of soufflé. French folks have a way of naming everything that is cooked brown in the oven a "gâteau."

Take one half pound of rice, wash it well, and put it into a pan with enough milk to cover it, with the rind of a lemon, and salt to taste. Let it simmer very gently till it has cooked itself into a soft, thick paste. You may add a little more milk from time to time, but don't let the mixture be sloppy at all; there must be no liquid in it when it is done. Take out the lemon rind, let the rice cool till you can hold your finger in it, and then beat in, one after another, the yolks of four eggs. Now taste again, and add as much salt as is necessary, with a dash of red pepper.

"Somebody once told me to put a very little mustard —" murmured the Story-teller.

"A fool!" was Colette's prompt comment. "Mustard with milk? *Mon Dieu!*"

"You are right," said the Story-teller meekly. "Go on."

"Butter a mold thickly — a tin mold is better than a china one — and sprinkle it with the finest browned crumbs. Beat up the whites of the eggs to the stiffest possible froth, fold them gently into the rice, fill the mold not more than half full — because the gâteau rises a great deal — and bake it in an oven brisk enough to brown it well, for three quarters of an hour. Turn out and serve immediately, before it has time to fall.

"Hand with it any sauce you like. Tomato sauce is delicious with it, and so is the Sauce aux Fines Herbes, which I gave you a little way back."

Now I want to tell you, if I may, a few of the more everyday egg dishes, those that Colette gives me when the Storyteller *isn't* here. They are very good, too, in their humble way, and much more quickly done than those elaborate affairs.

ŒUFS AU MIROIR (LOOKING-GLASS EGGS). Melt a little butter in an *au gratin* dish. Break in the eggs, two or three for each person. Sprinkle them with salt and pepper. Pour in a tablespoonful of cream for each egg. Slip the dish into the oven till the whites are *just* set. Have ready a browning iron and pass it over the surface to give a touch of brown. But don't make the eggs hard, or they will be spoiled. Serve at once.

ŒUFS AU BEURRE NOIR (BLACK BUTTER EGGS). Take two eggs for each person. Choose a frying pan large enough to hold them all at once. Melt a little of the best butter in it, heat the butter to spluttering point, and then break in the eggs at such a distance apart that their whites just join up, and all are attached together in a big sheet. Fry till they are set, the more lightly set the better, so long as the whites will hold. Slip them out on to a round dish without separating them.

Put into the frying pan another teaspoonful of butter for each egg, with plenty of pepper and salt. Heat fast till the butter stops spluttering and begins to brown. Then add one half teaspoonful of vinegar for each egg. Reheat again, pour quickly into the dish, and serve at once.

ŒUFS À LA TRIPE (TRIPE EGGS). Slice two large onions into a stewpan, with a piece of butter the size of an egg. Stand the pan beside the fire, and cook quite gently, till the onions are tender, but not browned in the least. Add pepper, salt, a cupful of cream, and a heaped tablespoonful of flour. Stir till it thickens, and then add one half teaspoonful of powdered sugar and from four to six eggs, hard-boiled, and cut into quarters. Cover the pan, and stand it where it will just keep hot — but will not boil — till the eggs are warmed through. Then serve.

"And omelettes, Colette, — what about those? A little while ago, I wrote 'cook the omelette in the usual way.' But there may be some folks who are not quite sure what the usual way is, you know."

"It is true, especially as there are two ways, the way of a Plain Omelette, and that of a Soufflé Omelette."

A PLAIN OMELETTE. Allow two eggs, one tablespoonful of milk, salt, pepper, and whatever seasoning you mean to use, for each person.

Beat the eggs, salt and pepper lightly in a basin till they are just mixed. Have ready a clean omelette pan, *which should never be used* for anything else. Melt in it enough fresh, unsalted butter to make it nice and slippy, but not enough to lie in a pond at the bottom. Heat the pan quite hot. Pour in the egg, which will at once begin to set round the sides. Keep the pan at a moderate heat, while you scrape the set sides of the egg into the middle, and allow fresh liquid to run out, and set in its turn. Do this till all the egg is set, but *not a second longer.* Flatten down the mass lightly with the back of a spoon, set the pan on the sharpest heat that you can get, and cook the omelette fiercely, while you count ten. Then slip a knife under and lift up a corner, just to see if the under side is brown. If it is, turn the omelette out, brown side up, on a hot dish, and serve at once.

If it is to be folded, with seasoning between, you must slip it out *brown side downwards.*

If you want to be economical, and make one egg do for each person, add, instead of the second egg, two tablespoonfuls of milk, with a small one half teaspoonful of cornstarch smoothed in it. Another very good plan is to use two tablespoonfuls of white crumbs, soaked in enough milk to cover them for one hour beforehand, and then beaten up well till they make a sort of paste.

SEASONINGS FOR OMELETTES

1. Pepper, salt, and the smallest possible pinch of sugar.
2. Pepper, salt, a small onion grated so fine that it is in pulp; a teaspoonful of chopped parsley, mint, and sage.
3. Pepper, salt, asparagus points, well boiled and drained, a tiny pinch of sugar.
4. Pepper, salt, green peas boiled and drained, just one little rub from a bead of cut garlic round the inside of the pan, before you melt the butter.
5. A very nice, thick purée of spinach or sorrel, spread on a hot dish, with a plain salt and pepper omelette laid on top.
6. Make a plain salt and pepper omelette, and turn it out pale side upwards. Sprinkle it liberally with grated cheese, and pass a browning iron over it till the cheese is very lightly colored. Fold and serve. You must never stir up cheese with the eggs and cook the whole lot together, or it will turn horribly stringy and indigestible.
7. Stir into the eggs before cooking a pinch each of red pepper and dry mustard, and a little lean boiled ham cut into wee dice, — about one tablespoonful for each egg.
8. Use pounded shrimps, or pounded salmon or lobster, with a dash of anchovy essence to deepen the taste. Dish such an omelette on a fish paper, and sprinkle it with chopped parsley.

SOUFFLÉ OMELETTES are mostly sweet ones, though you can also fill them with a savory paste, made of pounded shrimps or pounded game.

Take at least two eggs for each person. Separate the

whites from the yolks. Beat the whites to a froth so firm that a fork stuck into it will stand upright. In order to make the froth come up quick and well, you should

1. Keep in a cool place while you are whipping it.
2. Go always in the same direction.
3. Add a few grains of bicarbonate of soda. This helps it a lot.
4. Never do it till you are ready to use it. If you let it stand, it will be spoiled.

Mix the yolks just enough to break them up, adding a wee pinch of salt. Stir them lightly into the whites. Have ready your omelette pan, prepared as before. Pour in the egg, set the pan at once on a brisk heat, and fry sharply, *without any stirring or touching at all* till the bottom of the omelette is a good brown. Then take the pan off, and either hold it under a gas grill, or pass a browning iron over it, so that the top of the omelette, which is still quite raw, may get cooked. But *don't cook it too much:* you must not dry it up; it must remain so soft and fluffy that, when the omelette is folded, the fluff comes leaking out at the corners in tempting yellow foam.

Put in the filling, fold, and serve immediately. A Plain Omelette may, at a push, be kept waiting a few minutes, though it does not improve at all thereby: but a Soufflé Omelette must be eaten on the instant, or it will turn into a poor imitation of wet shoe leather.

FLAVORINGS FOR SOUFFLÉ OMELETTES

1. Jam of any kind, warmed till it is liquid enough to spread easily; or hot fruit purée, made as dry as jam.
2. Add a drop of vanilla flavoring to the eggs. Before you cook the upper side of the omelette, sprinkle it thickly with very fine white sugar.

Colette Cooks Eggs

3. Use any kind of savory paste filling that you like best. Warm it till it will spread easily.

If you want to cook eggs well, *always*

1. Break each one separately into a cup. Never mind how fresh it is. Even if you have heard your hen clucking, and have run out to fetch the hot egg she has just laid, break it into a cup first, all the same. There may be a " thread " in it that wants taking out, or one of those little red specks, which would spoil the look of any dish.

2. Never, if you can help it, cook eggs in anything but butter. Margarine, lard, butter substitutes are good for many things, but they ruin the delicate taste of eggs. Olive oil is the only alternative and that changes your dish, at once and forever. It is a nice dish, but the niceness is Italian, not French.

3. Keep a special pan for omelettes. If you use it for anything else — even once — you have only yourself to blame when the omelettes burn afterwards.

4. Remember that the less an egg is cooked, the more easy it is to digest, so, when you are making egg dishes for delicate folks, never let them go beyond the setting point, but take them away from the fire as soon as they have had the barest amount of cooking needed to make them palatable.

CHAPTER IV

FRENCH RAGOUTS AND STEWS

"COLETTE, I hear that they don't make good stews in America."

"*Tiens!* Why?"

"How can I say? Perhaps they don't know how. Perhaps, also, it is because they cook on gas stoves and electric stoves so very much, instead of on fires."

"I lived with a gas stove once," said Colette, in the voice of one who states that she has lived with a mad dog or a dangerous lunatic. "Oh, what misery I had with it! What an animal! It burnt all — all! But in the end I brought it to reason, and I made it cook quite well — even stews that need such a slow heat. Figure to yourself, I bought a big sheet of thin tin, just the size of the top of that animal. I put on the sheet of tin. I lighted one burner near the middle. All the tin heated itself, just as the top of my stove does — red hot near the burner, and cooler at the sides, just as the top of a stove is. I only had to pretend that there was a good little fire underneath instead of a gas, and then I was quite happy."

"It is an idea, certainly. I will tell them, over there, to try it. Now go on and tell them how to make some of your very best and most tender stews and ragouts."

RAGOÛT DE FOIES (RAGOUT OF CHICKEN LIVERS). Chicken livers are the nicest, but you may also use those of rabbits

French Ragouts and Stews

or ducks, if you like. Take out the gall bag, but leave the livers whole. Throw them into hot water, bring them up to the boil, count 100, and then drain off the water. Pour into the pan half a glass of white wine, with enough light stock to cover the livers; add pepper, salt, a good bunch of parsley, and a bead of garlic. Boil all for one fourth hour. Take out the livers. Arrange them on a hot dish. Skim the gravy carefully. Smooth one half teaspoonful of good corn flour in a few drops of cold water. Boil up the gravy again, add the corn flour, and stir till the sauce is well thickened. Pour it over the livers and decorate the dish with snippets of toast.

This is a nice little entrée or breakfast dish.

RAGOÛT DE CHAMPIGNONS (RAGOUT OF MUSHROOMS). Peel one pound of mushrooms, and put them into a stewpan, with two tablespoonfuls of butter, one tablespoonful of vinegar, one tablespoonful of chopped parsley, pepper, salt, and a good pinch of grated nutmeg. Stew gently for a quarter of an hour. Strain the sauce. Put the mushrooms on a hot dish. Reheat the sauce, and thicken it with one teaspoonful of corn flour, as directed above. There is no need to put any stock with this ragout, as the mushrooms give off a good deal of juice.

This is either a delicious breakfast dish, or it makes a nice lunch entrée.

CHOUX EN RAGOÛT (RAGOUT OF CABBAGE). Take the heart of a nice, firm cabbage. Throw it into boiling salt and water and cook it fast for half an hour. Then put it into cold water till it is cool enough to handle. Squeeze it well, to get out as much water as possible, and cut away the stalk. Chop the rest of the cabbage roughly. Now melt two tablespoonfuls of good beef dripping in a stewpan, toss the cabbage in it till well greased, and then sprinkle in two tablespoonfuls of flour, stirring well all the time. Add one and one half cupfuls of good, brown gravy, stir up well, cover the pan, and let it simmer very gently till the cabbage is quite tender. Season with pepper, salt, and grated nutmeg. Serve very hot indeed.

This may be served either as a vegetable or as a supper dish.

RAGOÛT MÊLÉ (RAGOUT OF LITTLE ROOTS). Take three each of carrots, parsnips, and turnips. Peel them, and cut them into neat little cubes or sticks. Melt three tablespoonfuls of dripping in a stewpan, and toss the vegetables in it till they are well greased. Take them out again. Stir one and one half tablespoonfuls of flour into what remains of the dripping, and, when it is smooth, add gradually one and one half cups of hot gravy, to make a good thick sauce. Return the vegetables to the pan, cover it, and simmer till they are quite tender. Add pepper and salt to taste, and one level teaspoonful of powdered sugar. Toss the vegetables well, so that the seasoning may be evenly distributed. Serve them in a hot dish, and sprinkle them with chopped parsley.

If you want to make a Ragoût Maigre, use potato water instead of gravy, and add a drop of browning to color it.

RAGOÛT DE GUERRE (RAGOUT OF POTATOES AND TINNED MEAT). We had this often during the war. Colette thought it one of the nicest ways of serving " box beef ", as she called the corned beef which came through to us now and then from America.

Melt in a stewpan two tablespoonfuls of the best fat you have; in the war we took what we could get, with thanks. Slice two onions into it and let them fry till they are lightly colored. Stir in one tablespoonful of flour and one pint of hot vegetable water or meat stock.

French Ragouts and Stews

Add pepper and salt. When the sauce has thickened, put in two pounds of potatoes, peeled and cut into moderate-sized pieces. Cover the pan and simmer very gently indeed, shaking the pan now and then, till the potatoes are almost cooked. Then cut one pound of corned beef or other pressed meat into little squares, add it, and simmer again till the potatoes are quite done. Turn all into a deep dish, and serve very hot.

This makes a good family dinner, — one that is very inexpensive and easy to prepare.

"Have you told them what slow simmering is?" asked anxious old Colette.

"Yes; I think so. But I'll say it again, if you like." When a thing is *simmering slowly*, the liquid in the pan must just move and bubble a very little, — ever so gently, and probably at one part of the pan only. But the solids in the pan — the meat and vegetables — *must not move at all*. If they dance about, the cooking is going much too fast, and the pan must be shifted to a cooler place. If there is no motion at all, the cooking is not going on, and the pan must be put a trifle nearer the central heat of the stove.

Always simmer with the lid on, because the lid keeps in the steam, and it is the action of the steam, almost as much as that of the hot liquid, which cooks the meat and vegetables.

BŒUF EN MIROTON. This is a stew of cold beef. Cold mutton, lamb, veal, or pork may also be arranged in the same way.

Melt two tablespoonfuls of dripping in a pan. Slice into it four onions, and let them cook very gently till they are tender and golden. Take care that they do not burn. Add one heaped tablespoonful of flour, and stir the pan over the fire till the flour is a nice golden color also. Then add one and one half teacupfuls of hot stock, stirring it in well, and pepper and salt to taste. Boil fast with the lid off the pan till the onion is quite tender, and only a tiny drop of sauce remains, just enough to cover the bottom of the pan. Then put in one pound or a little more of cold meat, cut into neat little slices. Stir them into the sauce, which will only just be sufficient to dampen them. Cover the pan and stand it at the side of the fire till the meat is heated through. Arrange the slices on a hot dish. Warm half a teacupful of vinegar in a little pan and trickle it over the dish.

This is a most delicious way of warming up meat. Colette wants you to notice with great care that the meat itself is never allowed to boil; it only stands beside the fire for just long enough to heat it through.

FILET DE BŒUF À LA SAUCE ORANGE (FILET OF BEEF WITH ORANGE SAUCE). Colette speaks of this with great respect; she says it gives itself at dinners of ceremony. It certainly is remarkably good. You can do much the same thing with a cheaper cut of beef, but that I leave to your inventive faculties to plan out.

Take a large tablespoonful of butter and roll it in as much flour, pepper, and salt as it can pick up. Put it into a saucepan and stir it while it melts. Then add the juice of two sweet oranges, salt, pepper (cayenne is best), and a laurel leaf. Add three quarters pound of mushrooms, peeled and cut up, and let the sauce simmer gently. Your beef should, by this time, have been roasted in the oven till it is half cooked. Now put it into the pot and stew it gently for half an hour, turning it so that all sides of it may get a little time in the sauce. Slice the beef thin. Arrange the slices at the center of the dish, put the mushrooms around, and pour the sauce over all.

French Ragouts and Stews

If you can't get mushrooms, use carrots, sliced thinly and boiled in salt and water for half an hour to make them tender, before they are added to the sauce; but you must prepare your mind for the fact that they will be a very second-rate kind of thing compared to the mushrooms.

BŒUF À LA FLAMANDE (RIBS OF BEEF, FLEMISH STYLE). Bone the ribs and beat them well. Roll and tie them in a neat shape. Put the piece of meat into a stewpan with three large slices of fat, salt pork or bacon, and let the beef fry in the pork fat, turning it constantly, till it is lightly colored all over. Then add half a glass of light stock, two laurel leaves, a sprig of thyme, and seven or eight little onions, neatly peeled. Cover the pan and let it simmer gently for three hours. Then add three large carrots, peeled, and cut into very thin rounds, and an onion stuck full of cloves. If necessary, add two or three tablespoonfuls more of white stock, just to keep the meat from sticking; but the less sauce there is with this the better. Cover the pan and stew very gently for three hours more. Then slice the meat thinly, arrange the slices in a dish, put the vegetables round as a garnish. Add half a cupful of boiling water to the pan, and boil it up on a clear fire, scraping the bottom well. Strain the sauce over the meat.

If you prefer, you may serve the whole joint on the dish, and carve it on the table. We never do this in France, but different countries have different habits, and there's no reason why you should not do it if you like.

BŒUF À LA PAYSANNE (COUNTRY BEEF). Take any cut of beef that has no bones — a lean piece of stewing beef is splendid for this purpose — and lard it thickly after having beaten it well with a rolling pin. Put it into a saucepan with water enough to cover it, pepper, salt, and a dozen or more of little onions, peeled. Let it cook very gently for six hours, turning it from time to time. Take out the onions. Leave the cover off the pot and boil as fast as ever you can, till the water is all boiled away and the beef sticks to the bottom of the pot and browns. (You may calculate that you ought to take the cover off the pot about one hour before you want to serve dinner.) Put back the onions and let them brown with the beef, turning both them and the meat, so that the whole affair gets well browned without being burned in any part at all. Now pour in one breakfast-cupful of water, just to detach the meat-juices from the bottom of the pan. Take out the meat. Slice it. Arrange it in the middle of a big dish and put the onions round it. Stir up the liquid in the pan very thoroughly indeed, and strain it over the beef.

This is a very economical stew, and a most delicious one.

BLANQUETTE DE VEAU (BLANQUETTE OF VEAL). Take two pounds of neck or breast of veal, and cut it into small neat pieces, leaving the bones. Throw the pieces into boiling water, and boil steadily for half an hour. Drain them. (Save the water for soup. It is very good.)

Now, in your stewpan, melt three tablespoonfuls of butter, and stir in two tablespoonfuls of flour. Let the mixture cook as much as it can, without getting in the least brown. Then add salt, pepper, and a little of the water in which the veal was boiled, till the mixture is thinned down to a nice, smooth sauce. Put in the meat, bring the pan to the boil, and then cover it, draw it to the side of the fire, and let it simmer for one hour.

Take out the meat, and put it on a hot dish. Beat the yolks of two eggs very thoroughly with the juice of a lemon. Add this to the sauce, return to the fire, and stir most carefully till it begins to thicken. Then take the pan off, add enough chopped parsley to look pretty, and pour the sauce

French Ragouts and Stews

over the meat. It should be thick enough to cling to the pieces and coat them.

A Blanquette Sauce, made with a little water or light stock, is excellent for reheating cold white meat of any kind, — rabbit and chicken, as well as veal.

POITRINE DE VEAU À LA POULETTE (BREAST OF VEAL À LA POULETTE). Cut a breast of veal into small neat pieces and beat them a little to make them tender. Put two tablespoonfuls of butter or lard in a stewpan. Let the fat melt, and then stir in two tablespoonfuls of flour, taking great care that it does not brown. Mix very well with water, to make a thick sauce. Put in the meat. Add pepper, salt, and a grating of nutmeg. Cover the pan and let it stew gently for one hour. At the end of that time, add one dozen peeled shallots, cover the pan again, and simmer for one and a half hours. Try the onions. If they are cooked, take out the meat. Arrange it at the middle of a dish. Arrange the onions round. Add three tablespoonfuls of thick cream to the sauce, stir well, and pour all over the dish.

This is very delicious indeed; — just the thing to form the main dish at one of your smart little lunch parties.

FILET DE VEAU AU JUS (FILET OF VEAL IN GRAVY). Choose a thin filet. Beat it well and dust it with flour. Melt three tablespoonfuls of butter in a large, flat stewpan and fry the filet in it till it is well colored at both sides. Now pour in a cupful of stock or water. Add pepper, salt, two lumps of sugar, and two cloves, with one laurel leaf. Cover the pan and put it into an oven hot enough to keep it simmering well. Leave it for one and a half hours.

It is a very good plan to cook potatoes with this meat, as they take the taste of it and become perfectly delicious. Choose smallish ones. Peel them. Put them into the pan at the same time as the meat, making a circle round it, and pushing them well down into the sauce.

When the meat is cooked, slice it thinly. Serve the potatoes on a separate dish. Put the pan on top of a bright fire, pour in a teacupful of water, and stir very well, so that you may scrape off whatever has stuck to the bottom of the pan. Strain the gravy over the meat before serving.

FOIE DE VEAU À L'ITALIENNE (CALF'S LIVER WITH MACARONI). Cut the liver into neat thin slices, and fry them lightly in a little butter in the stewpan. Add water enough to cover them, salt, pepper, six nice little onions, and a tablespoonful of cranberry or red currant jelly. Cover the pan and stew for three quarters of an hour.

Meanwhile boil a little macaroni in *plain* water, — a quarter pound of macaroni to each pound of liver. (The cook books — and their name is legion — which tell you to boil macaroni in salted water are obviously written by folks who have never even tried it, for salt turns macaroni hard in the boiling, just as it does beans. Salt should be added during the last five minutes, so that it may have time to flavor the sticks, but not time to harden them.)

Drain the macaroni. Take out the bits of liver, and arrange them on a hot dish. Simmer the macaroni in the sauce for ten minutes, and then put it around as a border.

Kidneys done in this way are ever so good. But they want a little drop of mushroom ketchup with them, in place of the jelly.

GIGOT À LA BONNE FEMME (STEWED LEG OF MUTTON). Melt three tablespoonfuls of good dripping in the stewpan, and fry the leg of mutton in it, turning it frequently, till it is nicely colored all over. Add one pint of water, pepper, salt, two laurel leaves, and a sprig of thyme. Under the leg of mutton in the pan lay a big slice of fat bacon or

French Ragouts and Stews

fat salt pork. Cover the pan and stew gently, but not too slowly, for five hours. At the same time, boil a good pan of haricot beans in plain water.

"Do they know that salt in the water turns haricot beans hard?" asked Colette.

"I have just said so. But we may just as well mention it, again." Well, strain your beans. Add a good handful of salt and toss them thoroughly in it. Make a bed of them on a big dish and pour all the mutton gravy over it. Then slice the mutton thinly and arrange it on top.

You can make a bed of mashed potatoes, if you like, but the haricots are more really French. They must be boiled till they are all broken and coming out of their skins.

FILET À LA FRANÇAISE (FILET OF MUTTON WITH FRENCH BEANS). Beat the filet well, fry it lightly on both sides in a little dripping, add a big cupful of water, pepper, salt, and two laurel leaves. Cover the pan and stew for two hours. Then skim off most of the fat, and put in one to one and a half pounds of nice little French beans, which have been already boiled for five minutes in salt and water. Let them stew with the mutton till they are tender. Serve them as a border around it. This is an excellent stew, though such a very simple one.

If you have a piece of rather underdone roast mutton, you may very well warm it up in this way, putting in the beans at the start, and stewing both together till the beans are cooked.

If the gravy is not quite as brown as you would like, add a drop of coloring.

HARICOT DE MOUTON (HARICOT OF MUTTON). Take about a half a dozen big turnips, and cut each into four or five neat pieces. Melt three tablespoonfuls of bacon or pork

Colette's Best Recipes

fat in a big stewpan. Now trim the cutlets of a neck of mutton, taking away most of their fats, which can be melted down and used for other things. If you are quite *en famille*, you may also use the lumpy little bones in the worst end of the neck, but this will not do for any smart occasion.

"A haricot of mutton does not generally appear in big dinners, does it?" asked I.

"Of course not. It is a dish that I serve to *you*," said Colette witheringly.

Fry the chops in the fat till they are lightly colored. Take them out. Fry the turnips also. Take them out. Thicken what remains of the fat with two tablespoonfuls of flour, letting it brown nicely. Add pepper and salt to taste and return the chops. Stew them gently for one hour. Now put in the turnips, making a sort of groundwork of them all around the edge of the pan, with the meat pushed into the middle. Peel a dozen and a half smallish potatoes and lay them on the turnips. Don't let them go down into the sauce; they are to be cooked in the steam only. Cover the pan and simmer gently again till the potatoes are tender (about one and a half hours). Stand up the cutlets at the center of the dish and make a border of vegetables. Pour the sauce over all.

PIGEONS À LA . . . I swept my fingers across all the keys of the typewriter at a swoop and then snapped them under Colette's astonished nose.

"If you think that, with that level, unexcited voice, which makes no change when the subject changes, you are going to slip along into the endless regions of game and poultry, my friend, you mistake yourself pretty thoroughly!" said I. "To-morrow, if you like. For to-day. . . . Fini!"

French Ragouts and Stews

If you want to make good stews, *always*

1. Cook them slowly.
2. Cook them too much, rather than too little.
3. Keep the pan covered all the while, unless you actually want to make the gravy boil dry. If you keep the lid off, the goodness of the meat goes off in steam.
4. Use only just as much liquid as is necessary to keep the things from sticking. If you put in too much, you will get a result which is neither quite boiling nor quite stewing.
5. When making the sauce, remember that it will thin out as time goes on and the juices of the meat run into it.
6. If the finished stew has sufficient fat to float on top of the sauce, skim it off. And save it for frying potatoes and other vegetables. It makes them quite delicious, because of the rich, meaty taste which is in it.

CHAPTER V

COLETTE COOKS BIRDS AND BEASTS

THE cooking of every country has its limitations, — its weak points as well as its strong ones. And it would be sheer foolishness in me to try to maintain that the French can teach other countries anything about plain meat cookery, — plain roasts, plain grilled, and fried things. Quite between ourselves, I never get a slice of roast beef worth eating except when I go visiting in London. Many years of painful experience have taught me that the only roast Colette can do decently is horse.

During the war, there was a time when our meat supply in this part of the world failed completely. After a week or two of nothing at all, we were thankful when the municipal authorities opened a horse butcher's in the nearest town, and we were quite polite to the dark, acid-smelling meat, which we tactfully named "steak." We tried all sorts of experiments with it, and, at last, Colette arrived at a roast which was quite delicious, — more like roast venison than anything else in taste, and as tender as a chicken in texture. May I just tell you about it? Not for present use, of course: but you may have a war in your country before this book goes out of circulation.

"The good God guard them from it!" says Colette devoutly.

Amen. With all my heart.

Colette Cooks Birds and Beasts

As soon as your horse flesh comes from the shop, put it into a basin, pour a cupful of vinegar over it, sprinkle it well with salt and black pepper, and stand it in the cellar for three days, turning it in the vinegar each day. Drain it until it will drip no more. Stab it in a dozen places or so with a small knife, and into each slit slip a piece of sliced onion. Baste it with any fat that you can get; when a country's eating horse meat, there's generally a fat-famine going on, too, but horse *must* have something of the kind, as it never seems to grow any fat of its own.

Roast it in the usual way, starting it with a strong heat, so that it may brown attractively. After half an hour of roasting in a dry tin, add about one half of the vinegar that remains in the basin, and baste often with this.

The meat should be very well done, — so well that it does not "run red" when you thrust a skewer into it. Underdone horse meat is revolting.

Slice it thin. Make a good gravy with the liquid in the pan. Don't try to save dripping, for there will be none. Thicken the gravy a little, and add a drop of browning to it before you pour it over the meat.

Cold horse is splendid for hashes and minces of all kinds, but you must manage to add a little fresh fat to it, or it will be too crumby. A small amount of it, used with a little fresh fat, some sieved haricot beans, a thick flour sauce to dampen the whole, and a little grated onion or grated cheese for seasoning makes a dish of mince or rissoles which is not only very nourishing, but quite excellent.

But, apart from horse, I am going to skip right over the question of roasts, for I feel pretty sure most of you could teach us more about them than we can teach you.

"Get on to the *interesting* things, Colette — all those

Colette's Best Recipes

delicious fancy dishes of game and rabbit and so on, which you do so *beautifully*."

Colette sighs, but gives up. She never can stand against a compliment. So here come the interesting things.

LAPIN À LA CRÊME (CREAMED RABBIT). Wash a nice young rabbit and joint it neatly. Melt two tablespoonfuls of butter or very good dripping in a stewpan, toss the joints till they are well buttered but not in the least browned, and then pour in enough cold water to cover them. Add salt, pepper, two bay leaves, six small shallots into one of which two cloves are stuck. Cover the pan and stew gently for one and a half to three hours, according to the age of the rabbit. When the meat is nearly tender, take the lid off the pan and cook fast till the gravy is reduced to half its first amount. Remove the shallots and bay leaves. Now mix a teaspoonful of corn flour in a teacupful of good cream, pour it in, stir till you see that the pan is just on the verge of boiling, and then draw it aside and let it simmer for quarter of an hour more.

The sauce should be so thick that some of it clings to and coats the joints. Pile them neatly in a hot dish, pour what remains of the sauce around them, and sprinkle all with chopped parsley. Very good indeed.

If you have no cream, use milk. If you think the sauce rather poor with only milk in it, add the yolk of an egg after the meat has been taken out, and reheat the sauce, stirring it all the while, till the egg thickens; but don't let it boil, or it will turn.

LAPIN À LA PAYSANNE (COUNTRY RABBIT). Joint the rabbit, but do not wash it; on the contrary, save all the blood most carefully. Fry the joints in a little dripping till they begin to brown. Then add three large chopped onions and brown those also. Last of all, stir in a heaped

Colette Cooks Birds and Beasts

tablespoonful of flour, and, as soon as it has colored a little, add a teacupful of water, with salt and pepper to taste. Cover the pan and stew, as above, till the meat is nearly tender. Then add the blood, the same quantity of brown vinegar, and, as nearly as you can judge, the same quantity of currant jelly. Simmer for quarter of an hour more, and then serve. It is a rich dark stew, which seems more like hare than rabbit.

LAPIN EN PÂTÉ (JELLIED RABBIT). We have two kinds of pâtés in France, — the minced pâté, and the jellied one, which is made of chicken, veal, or rabbit, and is thought a much better and more delicate dish than the mince. Do you have pâté pots in America, fireproof jars with lids, neatly finished off so that they can come to the table, and looking more like English marmalade jars than anything else? If you can possibly get one, you had better do so, for then the pâté can remain in the thing in which it is cooked, and, if it does this, it will stay good for several days more than it would do if it were turned out.

Cut the rabbit into small pieces, for convenience in packing, but do not take away the bones. Soak the joints very thoroughly in salt and water, to remove as much of the blood as possible. Then pack them into the pâté pot, sprinkling each layer with salt and pepper. Put in a small bag containing sweet herbs, a couple of onions, and a couple of cloves. Fill up the pot with cold water and stand it in the oven, with the lid on, for the whole day.

When you take it out, you will find the meat so tender that you can pick it off the bones without any trouble. Take care, won't you, that little splinters of bone don't get left in by mistake; they are so dangerous, especially for children. While you are picking over the meat, have the gravy in a pan, boiling fast with the lid off.

Colette's Best Recipes

Repack the pot, arranging the pieces of meat as neatly as you can, and putting truffles or slices of hard-boiled egg in among them. Pour in the boiling gravy and set the whole thing, covered, in a hot part of the oven till it just comes up to the boil. Then stand it in a cool place to set.

It keeps an astonishingly long time, if your pantry is cool and dry, and the lid is always on the pot. I have known it to last, in winter, a full fortnight, and be as good on the fourteenth day as on the first.

Veal and chicken can be prepared in just the same way. Neck or breast of veal should be used, with all the fat taken away. If you can add a little lean bacon or ham, so much the better.

Colette is remarkably fond of keeping ancient old grandmothers of hens, because she says they teach the young mothers how to bring up their families well; and when the poor old dears are really past work of any kind, she turns them into

POULE AU RIZ (FOWL WITH RICE). Pluck, clean, and truss the hen. Put into a big pot three pints of water, two ounces of butter, one large onion, and a dozen peppercorns. Let the hen be well covered with the water, and boil her steadily for two to three hours, according to her antiquity.

Take her out and keep her warm. Strain the liquor. Add salt and a quarter pound well-washed rice. Boil the rice till it is quite tender, strain it out of the pot, make a bed of it in a hot dish. Carve the fowl and arrange the joints on the rice. Cover them with Sauce Jaune (page 136) made with the liquor from the pot. The liquor that is left over needs only the addition of a little broken bread or toast to make an excellent soup.

Colette Cooks Birds and Beasts

That is, I think, our simplest and most family-like way of cooking poultry; let me give you something a little more fanciful.

POULET FARCI À LA CRÊME (CHICKEN WITH CREAM STUFFING). Prepare your chicken and roast it rather lightly. It must not be completely cooked. Carve off the meat of the breast. Keep the rest of the bird warm. Mince the breast meat finely, and mix it with

1 teacupful white crumbs soaked in as much good cream as they can take up
3 ounces butter
1 quarter pound mushrooms, cut small and warmed in the butter till they begin to soften a little
pepper and salt, with a little chopped parsley
the yolks of two and a half eggs. (Keep the other half for decorating.)

Mix all into a soft and pliable *farci*, and mold it over the breastbone of the chicken, so that it represents the meat which has been cut away. Put the rest into the inside of the bird, like an ordinary stuffing. Brush over the molded breast with the yolk of the egg, scatter it thickly with crumbs, and put pieces of butter here and there. Then return the bird to a good oven for quarter of an hour or so, till the made-up breast is nicely browned.

Serve with brown gravy, like a roast chicken. A salad dressed with cream is the proper accompaniment of this dish.

POULET À LA PIÉMONTAISE (CHICKEN IN ANCHOVY CREAM). Put two and a half pints of good bouillon (see page 12) in a pan large enough to hold the chicken; add two laurel leaves and two ounces of butter. When all comes to the boil, put in the chicken, breast upwards, let it cook till it is quite tender. Then draw the pot aside and allow the chicken to cool half an hour in the liquor. Take out the chicken, drain it, and keep it in a warm place. Skim the liquor. Now melt one tablespoonful of butter in a small pan; add a tablespoonful of flour and thin out the mixture to a sauce with the liquor of the chicken; add one to two tablespoonfuls of anchovy sauce and plenty of cayenne pepper, and let all simmer beside the fire while you are carving the chicken. Pile the joints high in a dish, pour the hot anchovy sauce over them, and decorate all with little snippets of fried bread.

If you find it more convenient to use whole anchovies, take four to six of them and pound them well before putting them into the sauce.

POULET SAUTÉ À LA MARENGO. Take a nice fat chicken, carve it raw, and cut off the flesh from the bones in the most substantial strips that you can manage. Sprinkle it with pepper and salt. Put into a flat-bottomed pan two tablespoonfuls of butter and two of olive oil. Warm these, and then put in the pieces of chicken, and fry them lightly, turning them so that they may be done at all sides. When they are colored, cover the pan and put it in a hot oven for half an hour, so that the bird may be cooked through.

Take out the pan. Sprinkle a heaped teaspoonful of flour into the fat, and add half a pint of good stock. Stir all up and stand the pan on top of the fire, so that it may boil. Add half a pound chopped mushrooms, and, when they are tender, stir in one tablespoonful of chopped parsley and one tablespoonful of currant jelly. Taste just before serving and add more pepper if necessary; for this dish, to be correct, should have a decided peppery sting in it.

POULET SAUTÉ AUX CHAMPIGNONS (CHICKEN WITH MUSHROOMS) is done in just the same way, except that you must use all butter, no oil, and the juice of a lemon must be added at the last moment instead of the jelly. Garnish the dish

Colette Cooks Birds and Beasts

liberally with little snippets of bread, fried very brown and crisp in butter.

POULET SAUCE BÂTARDE. This is a rather extravagant, but very delicious form of chicken in cream sauce. It is a dish to be served at lunch or dinner, when you have visitors.

Put into a pan large enough to hold the chicken two pints of bouillon, two tablespoonfuls of butter, a large onion, peeled and cut up, and a good bunch of parsley. Put in the chicken, breast upwards, when the contents of the pan have come to the boil; cook very slowly, basting often with the liquor, if there is not enough to cover the bird. Take out the bird when cooked and keep it warm. Boil the liquor fast, with the lid off the pan, till it is reduced to a quarter of its first amount.

Now roll two ounces of butter in one tablespoonful of flour. Bring one pint of good cream to the boil, add the butter and flour, and stir all till the mixture thickens. Then strain in some of the reduced liquor of the chicken.

Cut up the bird. Remove all skin. Reheat the joints in the liquor, which should be thick enough to cling to them and coat them. Serve with a garnish of green peas or asparagus points.

PIGEONS EN COMPOTE (STEWED PIGEONS). Allow half of a large pigeon for each person, and six little onions to each pigeon.

Melt in your stewpan a tablespoonful of butter for each pigeon. Brown them nicely in it. When they are well colored all over, add half a teaspoonful flour for each pigeon, pepper, salt, a bunch of sweet herbs, and enough water to cover them halfway as they lie in the pan. Fry the onions in a little butter in an open frying pan, and, when they are nicely colored, make a ring of them all around the pigeons. Cover the pan and simmer gently, basting often, till the birds are cooked, — three quarters to one and a half hours, according to size and age. Dress the pigeons at the middle of a dish, make a ring of onions around, and strain the sauce over all.

Practically all small game birds can be cooked in this way, though those which have a high and strong taste of their own do not need any onion. When no onion is used, serve jelly with the bird.

PIGEONS À LA CHIPOLATA. This is delicious, — one of those queer, mixed dishes, in which every mouthful is different from the one before and nicer.

Allow two small sausages and ten chestnuts to each pigeon.

Cook the pigeons *en compote*, exactly as above. In the meanwhile, roast the nuts and sausages in the oven, till the former are soft and the latter brown. Peel the nuts. Cut the sausages into pieces about the size of the nuts, or a little bigger. About five minutes before the birds are done, put the nuts and sausages into the gravy, and let the whole affair simmer gently together. Dress the pigeons at the middle of a big dish, with a border of mixed surprises all round.

PIGEONS AU PETIT POIS. Allow a quarter pint of freshly shelled peas to each pigeon, instead of the onions. Cook as above. A pinch of sugar is a great improvement. If you want to make the dish very pretty indeed, add a few wee baby carrots to the peas.

FILETS DE CANARDS AUX ORANGES (FILETS OF DUCK WITH ORANGE). Colette always says that there is no good at all in sending a whole duck to table. There is nothing to eat on the legs and wings — at least, nothing to mention — so it is much better to keep them out in the kitchen and use them straight away for the soup.

When a duck has been roasted, she cuts off all the breast,

Colette Cooks Birds and Beasts

and divides it into about six neat filets, sometimes eight if the bird is a very big one. Then she takes the juice from the roasting tin and mixes it with any other stock she happens to have, till she gets about three quarters of a pint of liquid. She thickens this with a very little brown *roux* and adds pepper, salt, and the juice of a lemon. Into this sauce she puts the filets of duck and lets them simmer gently for quarter of an hour, without ever coming to the boil.

Meanwhile, she peels an orange as thinly as possible, so as to get only the red skin, — no white at all. The red part she cuts into the thinnest of little strips — mere needles — and she boils these in plain water for ten minutes. Then she drains them well and mixes them into the sauce.

Between ourselves, I never can taste them; what I taste is the lemon. But they look ever so pretty and are quite a good change.

All water fowl may be served in this way.

Now, let us have just one or two veal dishes.

But first, just in case the same error may be current in America as in England, I had better ask you to notice two things:

Well-cooked veal is highly digestible.

Underdone veal is highly indigestible.

This explains why so many English say that veal does not agree with them. They cook it like beef — all pink — and it makes them ill; whereas, if they would cook it quite dry and white, it would suit them to perfection.

FRICANDEAU PARISIEN (PARIS FRICANDEAU). Take a nice veal cutlet weighing about two pounds. Lard it on one side only. Put into a saucepan

2 tablespoonfuls good bouillon
1 laurel leaf
1 onion with a clove stuck into it

Salt and pepper
The meat, with the larded side upwards

Cover the pan and set it to simmer for one hour, looking now and then to see that the meat is not sticking.

The larded side, which will not have been covered by the small amount of liquid, will remain uncooked, with melted lard running into all the holes and corners of it. When the hour is finished, uncover the pan, set it in a brisk oven with a good top heat, and brown the meat. Baste it often. It ought to become a beautiful deep brown. At the end of ten minutes or so, take it out, put it in a hot dish, and strain the gravy over it.

A fricandeau has all the tenderness of a stew, combined with the nice crispness of a roast.

CÔTELETTES DE VEAU SAUTÉES AU NATUREL. Use an open frying pan. Melt in it enough butter to cover the bottom, and fry the cutlets on a moderate heat, turning and moving them often, so that they may not burn. When they are firm to the touch they are done.

Now pour into the pan two tablespoonfuls of vegetable or meat boilings for each cutlet. If you have onion water or celery water, these are very good indeed. Add salt and pepper and enough brown *roux* to thicken the sauce. Let it boil up just once and then add a squeeze of lemon juice and a little chopped parsley. Arrange the cutlets on a dish and pour the sauce over.

This is one way of doing things. Another is to take the cutlets out as soon as they are fried, make the gravy afterwards, and pour it around them in the dish instead of over them.

VARIATIONS. 1. Fry a few mushrooms with the cutlets. Allow them about five minutes of simmering in the sauce before you serve it.

2. Use truffles cut into fine strips, instead of the mush-

rooms. Leave out the parsley and add almost nothing of lemon.

3. Use a little Sauce Piquante (see page 132) instead of anything else. No other seasoning at all, of course.

4. Brush the cutlets over with egg, dip them in crumbs, and fry them. Take them out of the pan. Decorate the ends of their bones with wee paper frills and stand them up in the dish. Add to the juice in the pan a little good meat essence or bouillon — about a teacupful — in which three grated shallots have been boiled. When the shallots are quite cooked, strain this liquor into the frying pan with the meat juice; add pepper, salt, and coloring; reheat to boiling point and pour around the cutlets.

CÔTELETTES À LA FLAMANDE. Fry the cutlets in a stewpan, — not in a frying pan. When they are well browned on both sides, pour in one pint of water or stock, and add one tablespoonful each of chopped onion and parsley. Put the stewpan into a hot oven and keep basting the meat during fifteen minutes. It should turn a very rich, dark color. Smooth half a teaspoonful cornstarch in a few drops of cold water, stir it in, and allow all to cook on top of the fire for five minutes. Then add pepper, salt, the juice of a lemon. Serve very hot indeed.

CERVELLE AU BEURRE NOIR (BRAINS IN BLACK BUTTER). Take off the thin skin with care and wash the brains well in several waters. When they are quite white, boil them gently for twenty minutes in water to which you have added salt, a dash of vinegar, a bunch of sweet herbs, and a cut onion. Drain the brains very well, keeping them warm all the while.

Melt three ounces of butter in a frying pan and cook it so fast that it browns. As soon as it changes color, add two tablespoonfuls of vinegar, with salt and plenty of pepper. Let all heat to boiling point. Pour over the brains, and, if you like, sprinkle them with chopped parsley.

RIS DE VEAU À LA POULETTE (SWEETBREAD À LA POULETTE). Sweetbreads must always be soaked in salt and water for at least two hours before use. When boiling, they should be quite covered with the water or bouillon in the pot, in order to keep them white. Do not cook them too long; twenty-five to thirty minutes is enough.

Prepare the sweetbread and boil it twenty minutes only. Drain it. Cut it into small cubes.

Put into a small pan a teacupful of the liquor for each sweetbread. Thicken slightly with white *roux*. Add salt, plenty of red pepper, a little chopped parsley. Add the chopped sweetbread and bring all to the boil. Then draw the pan aside, let it cool for three minutes, and stir in the yolks of one or two eggs, beaten up with the juice of a lemon. Return the pan to the fire, stirring all the while, till the eggs "take." This sauce should be very thick and clinging and should coat the pieces of sweetbread completely.

Ris de Veau may be served in almost any sauce you like to name, all made in a manner similar to the above. The nicest, I think, are:

1. Mushrooms stewed with the sweetbread and chopped up with it. No lemon in the sauce; and the egg is not indispensable, though it is, without doubt, a great improvement.

2. Green peas and a sprig of mint stewed with the sweetbread. Drain them all out. Make a plain sauce with one egg and a wee pinch of sugar. Not much pepper, and no lemon. Return the peas and sweetbreads together.

Colette Cooks Birds and Beasts

This sauce may be a little thinner than the others, and it is usual to trim the dish with snips of fried bread.

3. A little tomato sauce may be used. In this case, no egg is wanted. A couple of little onions should be stewed with the sweetbread, and removed afterwards. Lots of pepper, please.

PAIN DE RIS DE VEAU (SWEETBREAD SAUSAGE). This is a most excellent way of using up cold sweetbread. Measure your sweetbread and take the same bulk [of each of the following:

    Cold lean veal, pork, chicken, or rabbit
    Sausage meat
    White of bread

Don't mince the sweetbread; cut it into dice. Mix all well, with salt and pepper to taste, and either one or two eggs, according to the amount of meat that you have. Roll it into a long thin sausage, put a rasher of fat bacon on top, and bake in a moderate oven for twenty-five minutes. If you see that it is browning too much, lay on a second rasher at the end of a quarter of an hour or so.

This may very well be eaten hot, with any sauce you like. But I prefer it cold, with a salad and a nice little mayonnaise dressing; then it is quite delicious.

ROGNONS DE MOUTON À LA BROCHETTE (SKEWERED KIDNEYS). Plunge the kidneys into warm salt and water for a few minutes. Then skin them, clean them, and open them without separating the two sides. Thread them on a skewer of wood or silver (never of any other metal). Sprinkle them with salt, pepper, and olive oil and grill them on a quick fire. When they are done, unthread them. Lay on each kidney a little ball of butter, the size of a walnut, into which you have worked a drop of lemon juice and enough chopped parsley to make it pretty. Serve on a very hot dish.

MUTTON CUTLETS. See all the recipes for Veal Cutlets. Colette often gives me, also

CÔTELETTES DE MOUTON À LA SOUBISE. Fry the cutlets in egg and crumbs. Boil beforehand two small onions for each cutlet. Drain them, sieve them, and make a mound of the purée at the middle of the dish. Arrange the cutlets around it, with their frilled bones all pointing to the center. Into the frying pan where the cutlets were cooked put a little good brown gravy, well seasoned. Reheat this, with the fat that remains in the pan. When very hot, trickle it over the mound of purée at the middle of the dish.

Another of our war experiences made us very clever with tough beef, which, for many long months, was the only alternative to horse that we had.

IRON-POT BEEF. Don't waste a good cut in this way. But it is just ideal for meat that would otherwise be tough.

When the meat comes from the butcher, put it into a basin, pour a cupful of vinegar over it, and add black pepper, plenty of chopped sweet herbs, chopped onion or, better still, garlic.

Let the whole thing stand four days, turning it daily. Or, if you are in a hurry, you can warm the vinegar and seasonings, pour them on the meat, let them cool, and repeat the process. When all has cooled for the second time, the meat will be ready to use.

Take an iron pot, which can stand in the oven, and make in it a little thick sauce with dripping, flour, and water. There should be enough sauce to cover the bottom of the pan to the depth of two inches. Put in the meat. Add salt, pepper, chopped onions, and carrots. Cover the pot and stand it in a good oven to stew. When the lid heats, the top of the meat will brown. Keep turning the meat till it is browned on all sides. Then add a little of the vinegar in which it was soaked and let it simmer till, by trying it with a skewer, you find that it is perfectly tender. Slice it and strain the sauce over it.

This sauce should be about khaki-colored,—not very brown. You will find the flavor extremely good and the meat so tender that it will be difficult to carve neatly.

FILETS À LA SULTANE. Filet is the piece of beef that, in England, is called the undercut, the best and most expensive piece of beef that there is. If you wish to be a little more economical, you will find that a nice piece of steak does every bit as well.

Remove all fat, skin, and nerves from the meat, and cut it into neat little pieces about half an inch thick by three or four inches square. Sprinkle with salt and pepper and let them stand half an hour. Then mix together equal amounts of bread crumbs and grated cheese, roll the meat in this mixture, and fry the pieces in an open pan, using either butter or olive oil. When they are nicely browned at both sides, take them out and pile them up on a hot dish. Add a little thick tomato essence to the fat which remains in the pan, heat to boiling point, season with salt and red pepper, and pour around the meat.

I have never seen this dish served anywhere except in France. It is very good indeed. Those who are fond of onions may hash one and fry it with the beef, but the pieces must be drained carefully out of the fat before the tomato is added.

DESSERTE DE BOUILLI À LA FLAMANDE (FLEMISH BOILED BEEF). When a piece of beef has been used for bouillon and has been served plain afterwards, but has not been quite finished, you will find the following an excellent manner of warming it up again.

Melt three tablespoonfuls of good dripping in the stewpan. Slice in three large onions, and let them cook gently till they are clear but not in the least brown. Cut the remains of the beef into small, neat slices, roll them in flour, add them to the onions. Add just enough stock or water to keep the whole from sticking to the pan. Stand the pan, covered, at the side of the fire, where it will simmer along gently, without ever boiling. Leave it twenty minutes. Then add salt, pepper, a single large lump of sugar, and one and a half to three tablespoonfuls of vinegar. Taste well and increase the sugar if needed. Last of all, add a tablespoonful of fresh butter, and, as soon as this has melted into the gravy, turn all out on a hot dish and serve.

LANGUE DE BŒUF EN HOCHEPOT (TONGUE IN HOTCHPOT). Boil the tongue in a pot so large that the water will cover it well. About half an hour before it is done, add to it the following vegetables.

The heart of a firm cabbage, cut into four parts and blanched in boiling water.
Potatoes, carrots, and turnips — small ones, for choice — peeled but left whole. They should be about half cooked in salt and water.

Drain all the vegetables, put them into the pot with the tongue, and finish cooking all together.

Skin the tongue. Slice it thin. Make a ring of slices all around a large dish, piling them up like a wall. Drain the vegetables most carefully, and pile them as attractively as you can at the middle of the dish.

No sauce is served with this, and no other vegetable. It is a complete course in itself. The liquor is an excellent bouillon.

Colette Cooks Birds and Beasts

LANGUE DE BŒUF EN PARMESAN (TONGUE WITH CHEESE). Cut one pound of cold tongue into long, thin strips. Lay them in a dish which can go into the oven. Mix a cupful of good white sauce with half a cupful of grated cheese. Add a little pepper and a dash of mustard. Pour all over the tongue and set the dish in the oven till a little skin has formed. Sprinkle this skin thickly with grated cheese and a few white crumbs. Brown under a quick heat and serve.

Any meat can be done in this way, but tongue and ham are best.

HOCHEPOT DE PORC is made in just the same way as Hotchpot of Tongue, a nice piece of salt pork or bacon being used. But, in this second case, you need not limit yourself to the few vegetables that I gave you in the first recipe. Add also plenty of onions, a head of celery, and a good bunch of sweet herbs.

Reverse the order of arranging the dish. Pile the slices of meat at the center, and put the vegetables around the edge.

JAMBON (HAM). Perhaps you boil ham better than we do; I should not be at all astonished to hear so. But, just in case you might like a hint, I may as well tell you that Colette always rubs the ham all over with brown sugar the day before cooking it, and shakes all the sugar off again. Into the pot she puts enough water to cover the ham, and an onion stuck with three cloves and two tablespoonfuls of vinegar. She puts her ham into cold water, brings it slowly to the boil, boils it steadily till it is done, and then lets it cool in the water. Is that how you manage things, *chez vous?*

FROMAGE D'ITALIE (ITALIAN CHEESE) is not cheese at all, but a sort of cake of very rich cold sausage, most highly thought of in the south of France. It is very useful for picnics and such occasions. Serve it with salad.

Colette's Best Recipes

Chop and pound two pounds of pig's liver; chop, but do not pound, one pound of fresh bacon, not too lean; mix them with salt, pepper, mixed spice, and enough lemon juice to bind them into a paste. Line a plain round cake tin with thin slices of bacon; press the mince into it, cover with more bacon on top, and cook for an hour in a good oven.

Let the *fromage* get cold in the mold. Next day, dip it into boiling water, to make the fat on the outside melt; then it will slide out quite easily.

If you want to do good meat cooking, always

1. Buy good cuts of meat. The inferior cuts are not really economical, in the end, because they cook to waste, and give less soup and dripping than the good ones do.

2. Get your meat boned at the shop, or bone it yourself. If you attend to this, you will not only keep your soup pot always well supplied without extra cost, but you will save considerably on your fuel bills, for an unboned piece of meat cooks ever so much faster than a whole solid joint with a big bone down the middle.

3. Add salt towards the end of the cooking. Salt used on the meat at the start hardens it.

4. Keep trying all sorts of different sauces on boiled beef when it comes out of the soup pot. There are literally hundreds that are good with it. About nine tenths of the fancy meat dishes that you get in restaurants are nothing but boiled beef or mutton, sliced up prettily, dressed with a sauce, and called by a fine-sounding name.

5. Hang mutton. It wants to be *almost* high before it is really good. Use veal very fresh indeed, and beef moderately fresh. Cook rabbits while the life is still warm in them, but always leave chickens for a full day after killing, if you can manage it. They are eatable sooner, no doubt, but they taste of carnage!

CHAPTER VI

COLETTE AND THE LEFT-OVERS

"THEY don't have any," said Colette firmly.

"But, Colette, *every one* has left-overs!"

"Not rich people, like those Americans. Left-overs are for the poor, like you and me. I know it! Say no more!"

I said no more at the moment, but I was n't at all convinced that she was right. Folks may be as rich as they please, but they must eat left-overs now and then, all the same, for the simple fact that matter is indestructible, and that cold meats cannot vanish into air just at the will of the cook. So I hunted around in back numbers of American magazines and at last I found what I wanted in an advertisement, — a remarkably clever advertisement it was, too.

"Colette, look here!" cried I, swooping into the kitchen, magazine in hand. "You said they did n't eat left-overs in America. Well, they *do!* Here it is — printed — and with a picture! What do you think is in the dish that that pretty young lady is handing round? Hash, my friend, *hash!*"

Now, the French for mince is *hachis*, which is so much like *hash* that Colette recognized one word from the other. With her usual large-spiritedness, she gave up at once and began to take a lively interest in the left-overs, which she had previously sworn to be non-existent.

"Is it good *hachis*? Do they like it over there?" asked she.

Colette's Best Recipes

"Not much, I think. Folks in general don't seem to care much for hash and mince — except me. I like them always."

"That's because *I* make them for you," explained Colette, with perfectly innocent self-complacency. "A *hachis* is about the hardest thing there is to make — the thing that wants the most knowing how. Oh, yes! I know well that all cooks make it! But nine hundred and ninety-nine in a thousand make it wrong."

"Well! Tell me, then, how the thousandth does it."

"With thinking. That's what you must put into a *hachis* — lots of thinking. You must say to yourself: Here I am with a piece of meat which is cold

Cold	and must be	warmed
Rather dry	and must be	softened
Rather tasteless	and must be	made tasty
Probably not quite enough	and must be	helped out

And all this without being cooked again, because it is cooked already.

"I suppose it's no use telling those people to cut up their meat with a chopper on a board, instead of putting it through a food cutter, is it?"

"Considering the rate at which they live, I shouldn't think so. Why?"

"Because, you see, a food chopper, though good in many ways, squeezes the juices out of the meat and helps to rob it of taste. Also, of course, it wastes the meat a good deal, because some is bound to cling to the knives, even if one puts a bit of bread through afterwards, to clean them. But there! I can't insist: I leave it to their consciences!"

(So there you are, America, with a fine case of conscience to settle! Don't go into scruples over it, please!)

It is cut up — somehow — and, now, to each pound of

cold minced meat — weighed after all the bones and skin have been taken away — you must allow two ounces of something fresh and strong-tasting — something that has not been cooked.

If the hash is chicken, veal, or rabbit, use rather fat bacon.

If the hash is beef, use raw liver.

If the hash is mutton, use raw melt; or, if you can't get that, liver. But melt is best. Not more than a bare two ounces, it's such strong stuff.

The addition of the little scrap of fresh meat takes away all that toughness and stringiness — that shoe leather and cardboard feel in the mouth — which most folks dislike in minces and hashes.

Keep your raw meat separate from the cooked.

Melt a tablespoonful of butter in a stewpan, slice in an onion, and let it cook gently for ten minutes. Then take out the bits of onion with a fork. They will leave their flavor in the butter.

Put in the fresh meat, cut up small. Let it cook gently for five minutes. Then pour in enough stock or water to cover it, and add whatever seasoning you like. These are the ones I use:

If the hash is chicken, veal, or rabbit, a little mushroom ketchup or dried mushrooms, powdered; or a couple of sprigs of parsley and one leaf of sage; or six nasturtium seeds, tied up in a little bit of muslin, so that they can be taken out afterwards.

If the hash is beef, one teaspoonful of mixed spice to each two pounds with lots of salt, but no pepper; or two laurel leaves and two sprigs of parsley.

If the hash is mutton, a little tomato sauce; or one large tablespoonful of red currant jelly to each pound of meat.

Add the seasoning, — unless it is jelly, which must go

in at the last moment; or salt, which must also go in at the last moment, because it hardens the meat. Cover the pan; draw it to the side of the fire, and let it simmer gently for half an hour.

Now stir in the minced cold meat, which has been previously shaken up with one heaped tablespoonful of flour to each pound of meat. Return the pan to a good heat and stir fast with a wooden spoon till the hash *just* boils. Add a little more water, if necessary, to thin it out. For general purposes, it should not be thicker than whipped cream. As soon as ever it boils, draw the pan away, — it must not go on boiling, even for a moment, or the meat will harden. Let it stand at the side of the fire for quarter of an hour more, to warm it well through, and then serve it in one of the endless different ways in which *hachis* can be served. I'll tell you just a few.

ROSES BLANCHES (WHITE ROSES). Pour the mince into a large, heated dish. Have ready some hot mashed potato, made rather thick, and a large rose forcer. Force the potato in big white roses all round the edge of the dish. Put a little bit of parsley here and there, to make the green of the flowers. It's ever so pretty!

VIANDE AU GRATIN (MINCE AU GRATIN). Use, for preference, chicken, or some other white meat, and put no seasoning into it at all except the onion which is fried in the first butter, and a little pepper and salt. Pour the hot mince into an *au gratin* dish. Have ready equal quantities of crumbs and cheese, sifted together. Sprinkle them on top. Pass the dish under the gas griller, till it is nicely browned. This can be done in little scallop shells, too.

PAIN VIANDE (MEAT LOAF). Cut the top crust neatly off a new loaf. Scoop out all the white. Fill the loaf with nicely made mince. Put back the crust. Trickle gravy

Colette and the Left-overs

over the loaf till the crust is well soaked. Put it on a lightly greased tin in a quick oven and bake till the crust begins to brown. Serve hot, slicing it like a pie. It is every bit as good as a pie, for the soaked, baked crust turns crisp outside and is soft and meat-flavored inside.

When Colette does it for me, she uses a nice little crusty roll instead of a loaf, because, you see, a roll is plenty for one person alone.

HACHIS À LA MAYONNAISE (MOLDED MINCE). Add an extra tablespoonful of flour to each pound of mince, in order to make the hash a little firmer than it generally is. While hot, pour it into damped egg cups or tiny molds. When quite cold, loosen it with a knife, and turn out on a bed of small salad. Pour mayonnaise over all, and decorate with hard-boiled egg.

These are quite good substitutes for little aspics, if you have no time to do aspics. They would not be pretty enough for a dinner, Colette wishes you to understand; but "they are quite presentable for the family."

PÂTÉ. "This eats itself cold," as Colette says, and it is the handiest thing in the world for breakfast; for sandwiches; for pocket lunches; for any time when you want a slice of something cold to fill up the gaps.

When you are making your mince, add two tablespoonfuls of flour to each pound of meat. Don't thin out your mince at all, and don't cook it for the last quarter of an hour. As soon as it has just boiled up, turn it into a basin, beat the yolk of an egg into it, and, as soon as it is cool enough to touch, work it with your hands into a smooth, firm paste. It ought to be worked for ten minutes at least. Make this paste into a big sausage. Put it on a greased baking tin, brush it over with the white of the egg, sprinkle it with fine crumbs, and cook it in a moderate oven for half

Colette's Best Recipes

an hour. Don't let it brown, or it will be difficult to carve.

Let it get quite cold. Then slice it as thin as paper, and serve it with salad, pickles, or mayonnaise. With a salad border and a nice mayonnaise, it is quite good enough for an extra cold dish at lunch.

"One minute, Colette! You said you'd tell them how to make the mince go farther, if there wasn't enough."

"Yes, of course. There are many ways of doing it — all good."

1. When you are cooking the raw meat, add the same weight of crumbs as of raw meat, with enough liquid to cover both well, and boil them together. If bread is well cooked, it can't be either seen or tasted in the mince; it merely turns to a sort of jelly, which takes the meat flavor and rather improves the mince than otherwise. But you must not add crumbs without cooking them, or they will both taste and show. If it is possible to soak the bread in cold water overnight, so much the better.

2. Put hot, dry, freshly boiled potatoes through a potato press into the mince, and they improve it. But don't think, "I can use up a few cold potatoes in that mince," for cold potatoes are sticky and heavy, and will turn your meat into a sort of indigestible glue. Put the cold potatoes into the soup, if you like, but use fresh ones with the mince.

3. Boil a little rice in salt and water for at least two hours, till it is reduced to a soft, thick paste. Beat it up well with a fork and color it with browning before adding it to the meat. A little scrap of dripping, cooked with the rice, softens it and improves the flavor.

4. Freshly boiled haricot beans, mashed through a

Colette and the Left-overs

sieve, can very well be added to dry white meat, such as veal or rabbit. They make it drier still, and, so to say, intensify it. But you must not put them with a juicy meat, such as beef or mutton, or you will get a mince that tastes as if it had sand in it.

"And, now, Colette, supposing that they don't want mince, that they want to heat up the meat whole or in pieces; what shall they do?"

"Whatever sings to them the most sweetly — as long as they don't harden the meat. But they will — no doubt of that — they will!" Colette shook her head sadly. "However — ! Tell them they must first consider the piece of meat. If it is a boneless piece, which is rather underdone, this is a splendid way."

Make enough stiff mashed potatoes, mixed with pepper, salt, a little dripping and a little milk, to cover the meat with a layer about quarter of an inch thick. Smooth the potato on neatly with a knife. Brush it over with beaten egg and dredge with crumbs. Put it on a greased baking tin in a hot oven and bake it a nice, bright brown. Serve on a hot dish, with a little made gravy poured around. The potato and meat are carved and helped together, of course. The potato keeps the meat perfectly tender and prevents the juices from leaking out.

If there is a joint with a bone in it — a leg of mutton, for instance — the best thing to do is to warm it up in sauce. Make enough thick sauce to cover the bottom of a stewpan which will take the joint, and add vegetables, to flavor and decorate. These are the prettiest:

1. Stew some button mushrooms in the sauce. Serve them as a border around the meat, sprinkling them with a little chopped, hard-boiled egg.

2. Stew green peas and wee baby carrots together in the sauce. This makes a border "jardinière", which every one likes.

3. Peel little onions and stew them in the gravy, taking care that they do not break. When the meat is done, take it out. Leave the pan uncovered and let it boil fast, till the sauce becomes so thick that it sticks to the little onions and coats them. Arrange them in a border around the meat. Wash out the pan with a tiny drop of boiling water, to make just a spoonful of gravy, which you can pour over the meat. Those little onions — ah! Colette smacks her lips over them.

4. Boil some chestnuts for half an hour. Slip them out of their skins. Stew them in the sauce and dish them around the meat, just as you did the button mushrooms, taking care not to break them. They want rather a lot of salt and a wee pinch of mixed spice to flavor them.

5. Rub the skins off little new potatoes and stew them in the sauce. Dish them round the meat and sprinkle them with parsley and mint, chopped up together and mixed with the smallest possible grain of sifted sugar. There must not be so much sugar that you can see it — only so much that it brings out the taste of the mint.

Colette wants you to understand that meat which is cooked up in sauce must be stewed to rags. Visitors who go home from the Continent and talk about the meat cooked all to bits which they have eaten are talking about meat stewed up a second time in sauce. It's an extremely common dish in France, and every one knows, and takes for granted, that the meat itself will not be up to much; it's the sauce and the vegetables which will be so delicious, because they have all the juices of the meat in them.

If you want your warmed-up joint to be in nice, fresh

Colette and the Left-overs

slices, just as if it were newly roasted, you must *iron-pot* it.

If it is veal or lamb, squeeze the juice of a lemon over it first, to keep it white. Dark meats don't need this treatment. Spread a sheet of kitchen paper thickly with butter, wrap the joint completely up in it, and put it into an iron saucepan or stewpan, with a well-fitting cover. Put the pan into the oven. Our pans have no long handles, only little ears, like teapots, so they go in quite well. Let it stop till the pan is very, very hot all over. (A quarter of an hour in a brisk oven does it.) Take the pan out (and mind your fingers, please!) and set it at the side of the stove, where it will just hold the heat but not get any hotter. Leave it for a time varying from a quarter to three quarters of an hour, according to the size and thickness of the joint. It comes out of the iron pot exactly like a fresh roast. The well-fitting lid and the paper wrapping keep in all the steam, you see, and prevent the meat from drying, while the hot metal all around it warms it up to the right temperature.

You can't use any other pot than an iron one. No other metal can hold the right degree of heat. Some let the temperature drop too fast, while others get red-hot in the oven and spoil the meat.

Colette has a first-class way of warming up cold roast chicken, roast game, and roast rabbit. She gets the meat well warmed and yet not dried in the very least.

At the bottom of a saucepan she puts an upturned cake tin, so large that the chicken can sit on it. Into the pan she puts enough boiling water to come halfway up the tin. Then she covers the pan, puts it on a good heat, and lets it boil for half an hour. And then she carves her bird and

Colette's Best Recipes

serves it with fresh bread sauce and gravy. And even I, who am in the secret, can't always tell if the wing to which I help myself comes from a new friend or an old one!

It's a simple process of steaming up, of course. But I have tried the same thing in a steamer, and it didn't go. The bird was too far from the boiling water, perhaps. Anyway, he wasn't nice.

"Colette! Tell them how you turn the cold pork into turkey!"

"Do not talk foolishness! It is not really like a turkey — that is an illusion which you have."

But it's not. A leg of cold roast pork, warmed up in Colette's way, and served with a few fresh stuffing balls and some boiled and sieved chestnuts is, in my opinion, every bit as white and tender as the breast of a roast turkey. Try it and judge for yourselves. Only, please, don't take meat which is too much cooked; it should be rather underdone than otherwise.

Make a plain, short pie crust, using, if possible, some of the fat from the pork itself, — the dripping, you know, which came from the first roasting. Roll it out quite thin. Take all the crackling off the meat. Squeeze the juice of half a lemon over it, to keep it white. Wrap it up in the pastry, closing all the joinings most carefully. Bake it in a good oven till the crust is done. Break away the crust, and carve the pork, and serve it like turkey.

"The crust is for the kitchen dinner, or for the children, except when *you* — " says Colette severely to me "— come out here and spoil your good appetite by eating so much crust that you can't touch your meat afterwards."

I plead guilty. What else can she expect? That crust; with the pork and lemon juices in it, all hot and crisp, is quite irresistible. Of course, it can't make its appearance

Colette and the Left-overs

at a formal meal, because it breaks into untidy little bits when it is taken off the joint. But, if you follow my advice, you'll slip out into the kitchen and risk the wrath of your particular Colette, in order to get a taste of such a delectable "trimming."

If you want to do good left-overs always

1. Cook them as little as may be, unless you are doing meat stewed up in sauce. Then frankly cook it to rags.

2. Prepare the meat ever so carefully. Many a good dish has been spoiled by little scraps of skin and bone and fat, which had found their way into it.

3. If the meat is at all high, wash it in vinegar first.

4. If you use onions, mind they are well done. Little bits of hard, uncooked onion, mixed in with a dish of mince, are just about as dangerous to the digestion as so many little bits of glass would be.

5. Prepare only the amount you are going to want, in order to avoid the risk of having to warm things up a second time. Thrice-cooked meat isn't good for anything that I know of, — except, maybe, for helping folks to Heaven before their time.

CHAPTER VII

COLETTE AND THE CHAFING DISH

AT first Colette had a supreme contempt for the chafing dish. She called it "that toy", and absolutely insisted on my eating real meals, cooked in the kitchen, in addition to anything which it amused me to prepare in it. Under those circumstances, as you may readily understand, I soon gave up using it, and it stood on a high shelf of my sitting-room cupboard, waiting for its hour to come.

That hour was the time of the coal strike. We had not laid in our winter stock of coal, when, suddenly, there was none at all to be had, — not a lump for love or money. First we burned the little that was in the cellar; then we burned all our coke, and as much dry wood as the garden would produce. Then we bought a petrol stove at an exorbitant price, and it exploded and frightened Colette so horribly that I dared not try another. Then, at last, I remembered the chafing dish, sitting patiently in my cupboard, waiting to be used.

"It will explode," said Colette mistrustfully.

"Impossible!" I assured her. "Think of the many times I have played with it, and it has always behaved beautifully. It is made, you see, to stand on the table in a dining room — even on a table all set for lunch or supper. It is quite, quite different from that nasty petrol lamp."

Colette and the Chafing Dish

Colette took it gingerly between the tips of her fingers and retired with it to the kitchen, shutting the door firmly behind her. She and chafing dish were going to have things out between them. No audience wanted.

The result of that debate was such a supper as I had not tasted since the coal strike began. And, even now that the strike is over and she can burn as much coal as she wishes, Colette often lets her fire go out on a hot summer evening and gives me a chafing-dish supper. I like to watch her bending over it, with her old face puckered into absorbed wrinkles, and her squat, strong hands touching the dainty, shining little thing ever so gently. And her chafing-dish food is good! No doubt of that at all!

But I don't suppose that any of you are going to let your cook have the chafing dish to use out in the kitchen. You will be wanting to have it in the dining room and prepare your own little lunches or suppers on it, under the noses of your expectant guests. So perhaps you may be glad of just a hint or two, which will help you to save fuss and waste of time,— two things which are fatal to the success of a chafing-dish party. All the recipes in this chapter can be carried out on a gas ring or an electric grill, just as well as in a chafing dish.

Prepare beforehand, or have prepared in the kitchen, as much as possible of the foundation of each dish. Have fish washed, oysters cleaned, eggs hard-boiled (if that kind is wanted), cheese grated, parsley and cress washed, vegetables all prepared and put into cold water, toast made and kept warm in the oven till the last moment. It is a very good plan, also, to use tiny ramekin cases, either of paper or china as required, containing measured quantities of butter, milk, flour, and the like, so that you know exactly what you are taking without any trouble in weighing or measuring. Have all these things ready on a table so small that, when you have done with it, it can easily be moved aside.

It is a very good plan to keep at hand a small omelette pan, in addition to the regular frying pan. There are quite a number of dishes for which the one pan does not suffice.

There are certain things that seem to belong specially to the range of chafing-dish cookery, oysters, for instance, and eggs. I will tell you a few of the ways in which Colette does them, and you can invent others for yourself. One of the great charms of a chafing dish is that it lends itself so well to experiments.

HUÎTRES À LA CRÊME (OYSTERS IN ANCHOVY CREAM). *Prepare beforehand* one ounce fresh butter, well mixed with a teaspoonful of anchovy paste and a good dash of cayenne pepper

Five eggs, beaten up with a little salt

Twelve oysters, cut into neat dice

Twelve neat fingers of toast, buttered, and then spread with anchovy paste

At the moment melt the prepared butter in the blazer over the hot-water pan. Add the eggs and stir until the mixture starts to thicken. Then add the oysters, and stir again till the egg cakes around them, which it will do at the end of a minute or so.

Hand the upper part of the chafing dish around and offer the anchovy toast fingers with it.

VARIATIONS OF THE SAME DISH. Use half a pint of picked shrimps (measured after picking) instead of the oysters.

Use half a pint of neat flakes of white fish, previously cooked, instead of the oysters.

Use the fish as above, but do not take any anchovy at all. Instead of it, use one teaspoonful of lemon juice and

Colette and the Chafing Dish

plenty of cayenne pepper. Hand cheese biscuits or cheese straws instead of the anchovy fingers.

Use the white of a chicken, cut up into neat little cubes. Measure half a pint of them. If you want the real French flavor to this, rub the pan with a bead of cut garlic before you start and add half a teaspoonful of lemon juice to the sauce. Colette always puts salad on the table to eat with this, as chicken without salad would hardly be real chicken at all to French people.

HOMARD À LA DIABLE (RED-HOT LOBSTER). *Prepare beforehand* a medium-sized tin of lobster, finely chopped

One teacupful cold white sauce, rather thick

Little circles of white bread, stamped out with a cutter, fried crisp and brown, and kept very hot indeed till they are wanted

At the moment put the lobster and sauce into the pan and reheat, stirring carefully. Add salt, red pepper, one dessertspoonful made mustard, and one tablespoonful vinegar. When very hot, spread on the rounds of toast and serve, garnished with wee sprigs of parsley.

VARIATIONS OF THE SAME DISH. Any kind of white fish or white meat may be deviled in the same way. The fish should be broken up finely, or the meat minced.

Hot biscuits or buttered toast may be used instead of fried bread, if preferred.

RAGOÛT DE POULET AU RIZ (RAGOUT OF CHICKEN AND RICE).

Prepare beforehand one cupful rice cooked till it is just tender, but not at all squashy

One cupful cold chicken cut into large dice

One half cupful thick white sauce

At the moment rub the frying pan with a bead of garlic or a little cut onion. Melt a tiny piece of butter in it and

Colette's Best Recipes

just swirl it round, to make the sides slippy and prevent the ragout from sticking. Put in the chicken, rice, sauce, pepper, salt, and a good grate of nutmeg. Stir up well, cover the dish and let it simmer gently for twenty minutes. Stir it now and then and add a little drop of water or white sauce, if it is getting too thick.

Serve out of the pan. At the moment of serving, Colette generally produces from the kitchen a plateful of little wedges of crisp fried pastry, which she sticks in all around the dish to garnish it. They are ever so good with the creamy white ragout — they give just that little crackling in the mouth that is so nice — but, if they cannot conveniently be obtained, the dish can quite well be served without them.

VARIATIONS OF THE SAME DISH. Use half a cupful of cold veal and half a cupful of lean ham instead of the chicken. No nutmeg, but a laurel leaf simmered in the ragout and taken out before serving. I like this better than the chicken, myself.

You can do the same thing with mutton and a brown sauce, instead of white meat and a white sauce. But it is ordinary. Colette thinks nothing at all of it, even when it is flavored in the way I like best, with an onion stuck with two cloves. The onion comes out before the ragout is served, of course.

The remains of a boiled or stewed rabbit, with a sauce made of his own gravy, cook up into the most delicious ragout you can imagine. Add pepper and salt only as the first seasoning. But, just before serving, stir in a heaped tablespoonful of red currant jelly and a teaspoonful of brown vinegar. You wonder, then, whether you are eating rabbit or hare! But, anyway, you know that you have struck something mighty good.

Colette and the Chafing Dish

FOIE À LA MINUTE (HASTY LIVER). *Prepare beforehand* half a pound calf's liver, cut into neat thin slices, and rolled in flour, pepper, and salt

One peeled and chopped shallot

A little parsley

At the moment melt half an ounce of butter in the deep pan and fry the shallot in it. Put in the sliced liver and turn the pieces carefully with a fork, taking pains to keep them from burning, till they are neatly fried at both sides. Now add three tablespoonfuls of gravy or stock and the same amount of tomato sauce, with salt and red pepper to taste. Stir the pan till it comes up to the boil and then simmer for five minutes. Sprinkle with chopped parsley and serve from the pan.

Hand fried potato ribbons or chips with this, if you can manage it. They are a very great improvement to it.

VARIATIONS OF THE SAME DISH. Kidneys sliced and cooked like this are quite delicious. Season them with a few chopped mushrooms, or a little mushroom sauce, instead of the tomato.

PETITS POIS À LA FRANÇAISE (FRENCH PEAS). You can use preserved peas for this in winter, when no fresh ones are to be had. The dried ones, in packets, do just as well as bottled peas, and are cheaper.

Prepare beforehand one pint of peas, cooked, drained, and kept hot

One dessertspoonful chopped parsley

Put the peas into the deep pan with four tablespoonfuls of cream. It need not be double cream — a thin cream will do, though, of course, the thicker and richer cream you can get, the better the dish will be. Add pepper, salt, and half a teaspoonful powdered sugar, with a large sprig of fresh green mint. Stir carefully, never allowing the cream to come to the boil. This is most important; if it boils it is spoiled. When thoroughly hot, turn into a warmed vegetable dish and sprinkle with chopped parsley before serving.

VARIATIONS OF THE SAME DISH. If you can't get cream, or if you think it too costly, make a rather liquid white sauce with butter. It is almost as good. In this case, don't use powdered sugar, but take one big lump of cube sugar and rub it well on a cut onion before you put it in. The tiny touch of onion is very nice — it picks out the flavor of the peas — but you can only use it with sauce, — never with milk-cream.

SWISS RABBIT. "Rabbits that have no legs" seem to belong especially to chafing-dish cookery. You know lots of them already, I expect, for I have, at different times, eaten "Boston Rabbit" and "American Rabbit." But perhaps this one may not be known to you, and it is particularly nice and economical.

Prepare beforehand a fresh egg, beaten up in a cup with one ounce of crumbs and three tablespoonfuls of cream or "the top of the milk"

Three ounces of grated cheese — Gruyère is best, but nice dry Cheddar will do

Four nice little half-rounds of hot buttered toast

At the moment melt one ounce of butter in the chafing dish, put in all the other things, with lots of salt and pepper, and a dash of mustard if you like. Stir all over a good heat till the mixture is piping hot and quite smoothly mixed to a cream. Then pile it on the pieces of buttered toast.

A Swiss Rabbit, as a rule, is not very hot in flavor, so don't be too generous with your pepper and mustard.

VARIATIONS OF THE SAME DISH. "There are none," says

Colette and the Chafing Dish

Colette. "Every Rabbit is so different that each must have its own recipe."

"Well, I can't write more than one more, so pick out the nicest."

OLD ENGLISH RAREBIT. *Prepare beforehand* six ounces of Cheddar cheese, cut up into thin slices

Six nice half-rounds of buttered toast

At the moment put the cheese into the pan, with half a teaspoonful mustard and one quarter pint ale. Add red pepper to taste, but no salt. Stir over a sharp heat till the mixture becomes creamy, and then pour on to the toast and serve very hot indeed.

"But, Colette, I never tasted ale in my life, and I am sure I should not like it if I did!"

"Well, then, milk can be used instead of the ale. It is very good when done with milk, but a little salt is needed — just a wee pinch — to pick up the flavor."

ŒUFS À LA JARDINIÈRE (GARDEN EGGS). *Prepare beforehand* half a pint macedoine of vegetables (You can either use it cold, left over from a previous meal, or you can use the macedoine that comes bottled.)

Half a teacupful good white sauce

Four hard-boiled eggs, cut into slices

One small shallot, chopped finely

At the moment melt one ounce butter in the chafing dish, fry the shallot lightly in it, and, when it just begins to color, add the vegetables, and let them just color too. Then stir in the sauce and let all get thoroughly hot, taking care that nothing sticks to the pan. Last of all add the eggs and give a good shake-up, so that the eggs settle down among the vegetables. Serve piping hot from the pan.

Little triangles of fried bread, stuck in all round the dish at the moment of serving, are a great improvement.

Colette's Best Recipes

VARIATIONS OF THE SAME DISH. Half a dozen mushrooms, peeled, cut into little pieces, and fried in the butter, are even nicer than the onion, some folks think. If you cannot easily get a macedoine, take just one vegetable, or perhaps two — carrots and green peas are excellent together; or dried haricot beans alone make a dish which looks less pretty, but is very good indeed if you use plenty of onion and a sprinkling of mixed herbs,— parsley, mint, and thyme.

"Now, Colette, something with which to finish up the meal, please!"

DEVILED ALMONDS À L'ITALIEN. *Prepare beforehand* half a pound of almonds, blanched in boiling water, skinned, and then most carefully dried on a soft cloth

One saltspoonful of salt, cayenne, and curry powder, well mixed together

(Some like a little more salt and less pepper and curry)

At the moment put one large tablespoonful of the best sweet olive oil into the frying pan and let it get hot. Then add the almonds and fry them a good golden brown, tossing them often, so that the color may be even and clear. Pour off every drop of the oil, so that the almonds remain quite dry in the hot pan. Then add the salt mixture and stir them in it with your fingers, working and rubbing them till they are almost cold. Have ready a little silver dish or basket, lined with a lace paper. Turn them out into this and hand them with the coffee at the end of the meal.

"Why do you never cook sweets in my chafing dish, Colette? I should have thought it would be quite nice for fritters and so on."

"Because you have only one pan," answered Colette promptly. "And, as every clean cook knows, milk things or fruit juice must never, never be cooked in a pan that is used for meat or vegetables. You may say, as much as you like, that good washing takes away the taste of all previous dishes; but it is not true. Nine people out of ten will detect nothing; but the tenth will taste that there is something wrong. And, as you know very well, one must always cook for the tenth — the person with a palate. If one gets into the habit of cooking for the nine who taste nothing, in a few weeks one will be having complaints from the pigs because their mash is so badly made that they can't eat it."

Which is, I suppose, her eminently practical translation of the saying, "You must aim at the stars if you want to hit the chimney pots!"

CHAPTER VIII

COLETTE COOKS FISH

COLETTE has one sworn enemy, — the fish merchant. To me he seems to be a pleasant little fellow enough, with a smile that would be quite charming if his teeth were not so broken. But Colette hates the very sight of him, scolds at his wares, at his prices, at his manner of ringing at our gate, at his donkey's manner of nibbling the hedge while it waits, — in fact, at everything to do with him. Under the circumstances, it is hardly wonderful that he manages adroitly to trade off on her the smallest and boniest and least fresh of his fish. And whatever treatment it gets in the kitchen does n't help it much. So my Fridays are real seasons of penance.

It was on a Friday, after a particularly uneatable lunch, that I said gently to Colette that I thought I would go up to the convent on the hill, and ask the kitchen Sister to tell me something about cooking fish. "Because I don't think it is your strong point, is it?" said I. "And, of course, I want the best possible recipes to put in the book."

Oh, my goodness! Colette suddenly went hopping, dancing, shouting mad! Though whether she was blaming me, who was so difficult about my food: or the evil fish-peddler, who sold her such muck: or the Holy Father, who orders Friday abstinence: or Almighty God, who created "whales and all that move in the waters" is really more

Colette Cooks Fish

than I can tell you. Maybe it was the whole lot of us. She had indignation enough to go round, and leave a little over!

Well, well! It passed, as all storms do. And, in proof of her repentance for having made such a scene, Colette set to and gave me a number of most mouth-watering recipes for fish-cookery. She has kindly promised to do them all for me — when the fish merchant gets gaoled at last, and his place is taken by an honest man with decent wares.

I expect that it is the same all the world over; in the inland districts of big countries the folks are bound to go in for a good deal of salt fish. Salt cod is what we get, mostly: but any other kind of large salt fish would answer the same purpose.

All salt fish should be soaked in cold water overnight. If a strong salt taste is disliked, the fish should be put into cold water, brought to the boil, and then taken out before cooking. This process may be repeated once or even twice. If the fish is never allowed actually to boil, it will not lose anything of its food value.

MORUE AUX POMMES DE TERRE (COD WITH POTATOES). After preparing the fish as above, put it into cold water, bring it just to the boil, skim it, cover the pan and draw it aside, allowing the fish to cook gently for quarter of an hour. Then drain it out and keep it warm, while you cook in its water six large potatoes, peeled and cut into halves lengthwise. Drain them. Dish them around the fish and pour over all a nice cream sauce with a little parsley in it.

BRANDADE DE MORUE (BRANDADE OF COD). Boil the fish as above. Take away all the skin and bones and break the flesh into flakes. Put two tablespoonfuls of the best olive oil in a pan, add the fish, set the pan on a moderate heat, and stir constantly with a wooden spoon. When you see that the mixture is becoming too dry, add a very few drops of milk. Keep on doing this from time to time, stirring constantly, till the mixture becomes a soft, smooth paste (in about twenty minutes). Pepper it strongly. Pile it on a hot dish. Chop a couple of truffles and sprinkle them over it; but, whatever you do, don't put any parsley near it, not even for decoration, or you will spoil it completely.

MORUE À LA BOURGUIGNOTE. Boil the fish as above. In a pan large enough to hold the fish, make a pint or so of simple brown sauce. (Poor Man's Gravy does very well.) Peel twelve little onions and add them to the sauce, with pepper, salt, a good bunch of mixed herbs, and as much mixed spice as will lie on the nail of your least finger. Cover the pan and let the onions cook gently in the sauce. When they are almost done, put back the fish with them, and let it simmer for the last quarter hour.

Remove the bones and skin from the fish; arrange the flakes in a pile at the middle of a dish, put the onions around, and pour the sauce over all.

If the sauce has thinned down a little in the process of boiling, thicken it up with a teaspoonful of cornstarch, smoothed in a little drop of cold water. It should be thick enough to coat the fish and cling to it.

MORUE À LA MAÎTRE-D'HÔTEL. When your fish has been boiled, take away all the skin and bones and break the flesh into large flakes. In a flat dish melt a piece of butter the size of two eggs, and add to it a tablespoonful of vinegar, a little chopped parsley, a good pinch of coarse pepper, and a little grated nutmeg. Stir all well together. Stand the dish on the edge of the stove, where it will keep very hot, and turn the flakes in the sauce till they are buttered

Colette Cooks Fish

all over. Serve immediately. If you let the dish hang about in the oven, so that the fish dries up, it will be good for nothing at all.

There are two standard French ways of cooking unsalted boiled fish, which can be used for any kind you like, provided that it is large enough to be separated neatly from the bones and skin.

Boil your fish gently, so that it may not break too much. Take away the bones and skin and divide the flesh into large flakes. Put them on a hot dish and cover them either with SAUCE AU BEURRE NOIR (BLACK BUTTER) (see chapter on Meat Cookery) or SAUCE JAUNE (see chapter on Sauces). Fish water is used as the liquid of the sauce, and, as a rule, a sprinkling of parsley is added as a garnish to the finished dish.

If any of this large-flaked fish is left, the best way of warming it up is

BEIGNETS DE POISSON (FISH FRITTERS). Scrape away all the sauce. Put the flakes in a dish with salt, pepper, and a little vinegar, and leave them to soak for a couple of hours, so that they may be well seasoned. Then shake them very dry, dip them in Beer Batter (see article on Frying), and fry them in deep fat, heated to smoking point. Serve very hot, piled up on a dish and garnished with fried parsley.

If you don't care about fried things, perhaps you would prefer

POISSON AU GRATIN (FISH AU GRATIN). Melt a good piece of butter in an *au gratin* dish and sprinkle it with crumbs, pepper, and salt. Toss the fish in its own quantity of thick white sauce and put it in the dish. Cover it with more crumbs, add little bits of butter here and there, and brown it in a good oven.

Colette's Best Recipes

That is the respectable *au gratin*, which every one has. Personally, I think it dull, and very much prefer a

AU GRATIN FLAMANDE (FLEMISH HASHED FISH) which Colette says is "low", and will only give me when I am alone.

Mix together a cupful of crumbs and a cupful of chopped onions, and fry them in three tablespoonfuls of olive oil till they are a nice brown. Put a layer in the dish: then add the fish, turned in white sauce, as before; then another crisp brown layer to finish off; and just heat the whole thing well through in the oven.

Any one who is fond of onions will find it perfectly delicious. But, as Colette thinks it "low", I must not insist on it. Let us pass to higher subjects!

TROUT À LA GÉNEVOISE is a dish of which she quite approves. And it is very good, too.

Clean and scale the fish and put them on to boil gently in salt and water. After their water has begun to boil and has been skimmed, put in a large crust of bread, — the whole bottom of a loaf, probably, for four trout.

While the fish and bread are boiling, prepare the following sauce:

Melt in a saucepan a piece of butter about half the size of an egg. Add two chopped shallots, a tablespoonful of chopped parsely, salt, pepper, and six mushrooms, peeled and chopped. Take the piece of bread out of the fish pan — being careful not to break it — and, after it has drained for five minutes, add it to the sauce. It will suck up all the butter, and a great many of the seasonings will stick to it. After it has simmered for five minutes, lift it carefully to a hot dish, pile on it any seasonings that it has not absorbed, and finally add the boiled and well-drained fish. I have never seen this dish anywhere outside France.

Colette Cooks Fish

If, by bad luck, the crust should break, you must beat it all to a paste and put it through a sieve, making a sort of purée of it in the dish. This tastes all right, but it is a confession of failure, for, of course, the crust shouldn't break at all.

FRIED TROUT are served all the world over, and lots of folks do them well. But I wonder if any one else does them just as well as a woman with whom I once went camping? Her fried trout were really too good for this wicked world.

She cleaned them first, and dusted them with a little flour.

Then she filled her fry pan with the best olive oil to such a depth that the fish would just be covered.

She heated the oil till it smoked and then put the fish in.

She fried them *very much*, — almost to the verge of burning.

She sprinkled them with salt and red pepper before serving, and squeezed the juice of a lemon over them as they lay piled in the dish.

HERRINGS are very much eaten in France, and the one curious point about the manner of preparing them is that they are *never washed*. Colette would not even look at a herring that had been in water since it left the sea. They are emptied, wiped out with a bit of clean rag, and then carefully dusted with salt, pepper, and a grain or two of dry mustard before being either fried or grilled. If you use a grill — which, Colette says, is much better than a fry pan for such a greasy-fleshed fish — remember to make it *red hot*, and then the herrings won't stick to it.

HARENGS DE DIEPPE (DIEPPE HERRINGS). Take a dozen fine herrings, clean and scale them, and wipe them as dry as you can.

Colette's Best Recipes

Put on the fire a saucepan with

> ½ pint water
> ¼ pint vinegar
> The juice of 3 oranges
> 1 large onion, peeled and chopped
> 2 carrots
> 2 beads garlic
> 12 peppercorns
> A bunch of fresh sweet herbs

Cook all together for quarter of an hour. Put in the herrings. Let them boil for six minutes. Draw the pan off the fire and let them get cold in the water.

When they are perfectly cold, drain them well, pile them up on a fish paper, decorate them with parsley, and serve them with a cold cream sauce which contains a good deal of salt; for, as you may have noticed, no salt is cooked with the fish at all.

HARENGS EN SALADE (SALT HERRING AND POTATO SALAD). Open the salt herrings. Pour boiling water over them till the skin and bones become loosened. Then take away all that you can, dividing the flesh into neat filets. Make an ordinary potato salad, and trim it with the little pieces of fish, and with a couple of hard-boiled eggs, cut into slices.

FILETS DE MERLAN À L'ORLY (FILETS OF WHITING À L'ORLY). Colette says that medium whitings are the best. The little ones are nothing but skin and bone, while the big ones are apt to taste coarse. So take the filets of three medium whitings, split them down the middle, so that each fish yields four long thin pieces, and put these pieces into a dish, with the juice of a lemon, salt, pepper, and a couple of sprigs of parsley — whole, not chopped. Leave them to soak for at least two hours. Just before the meal, drain

Colette Cooks Fish

them, roll them in very finely sifted flour, and fry them in smoking hot oil, which is just deep enough to cover them.

They should be perfectly dry and crisp, more like pieces of biscuit than anything else. Pile them on a heated napkin and decorate them with fried parsley and slices of lemon.

SOLES in France are practically always cooked in white wine. The only exception that I know of is

FILET DE SOLE À LA BROCHETTE. Divide each filet, making two long, thin strips of it, and cut shadow-thin pieces of fat bacon just to fit them. Pound a little onion and pepper together in a mortar till you get a paste, which can be spread very thinly on the fish. Now lay a piece of bacon inside each piece of fish, roll them up together, pass them through flour. Slip a skewer through several little rolls at a time. Dip them into deep fat heated to smoking point, and fry them a good brown. Serve very hot indeed.

ROUGET À L'HUILE. (If you don't have those pretty, pink-splashed fish in America, you will find, I think, that a small fresh haddock cooks very well in the same fashion, though, of course, the flesh of a rouget is more delicate.)

Clean and wash the fish. Put on to boil

> 1 quart water
> 1 teacupful vinegar
> 2 peeled onions
> 2 peeled carrots
> Salt, pepper, a bunch of sweet herbs
> 1 tablespoonful butter

Boil all this for half an hour. Then empty and wash the fish and put it in. Rouget takes only a minute to cook: haddock much longer. When it is done, drain it out, let it get perfectly cold, and then serve it with oil and vinegar.

HUÎTRES (OYSTERS). "But you know that it is a crime to

cook oysters! All those who eat with intelligence, take their oysters raw — unless they want to play with them in that chafing-dish toy of yours," protests Colette. But I insist on a recipe or two, being myself sufficiently lacking in intelligence to prefer cooked oysters to raw ones.

There is one very good way of doing them, in which they remain really raw, but do not seem to be so, if you understand me.

Allow one small shallot and a tablespoonful of vinegar for each oyster. Pound the shallots in a mortar till they are reduced to pulp; then add the vinegar, and a liberal seasoning of black pepper, a little salt, and the merest shadow of fine sugar. The amount of sugar to be used is a very delicate matter, for none at all leaves the dish insipid, while even a little too much makes it uneatably nasty. Add it grain by grain, tasting all the time. Open the oysters and pour the sauce on each in its shell.

HUÎTRES AU NATUREL (GRILLED OYSTERS). Open large oysters. Place on each a piece of butter the size of a small nut, into which has been rolled a good allowance of chopped parsley, a big pinch each of salt and pepper, and a grain or two of mixed spice. Set the oysters on the grill. Take them off the moment they begin to boil, and serve them at once.

If you want to do good fish cooking *always*

1. Test whether boiled fish is done or not by slipping a fine skewer along the side of the backbone. If the least resistance is felt, the fish is not done yet.

2. Bring fish up to the boiling point very fast. Skim it. Draw it aside and let it simmer till it is done. Never let it boil hard after the skimming; this is the secret of keeping it both whole and of a good flavor.

3. Fry fish in oil whenever you can. It is one of my

Colette Cooks Fish

complaints against Colette that she *will* use dripping, which makes heavy, soggy fried fish, whereas oil makes it crisp and light and crackling. Olive oil does very well indeed, but still better is the cheap oil — called by no name that I have ever found out except just "oil" — which is used by the owners of fry stalls in gutters, and fried fish and chip shops in "mean streets." But it's hard to get, especially for those who shop in automobiles, or on the 'phone, and, as I said, the olive oil does quite well.

4. Never fry fish till the minute before you want to serve it. It should go straight from the pan to the table.

5. Be ever so careful in the preparation, — the removal of bones and skin, and so on. The fact that these things are often found so bothersome at table is the reason why many persons object to fish.

6. We never serve any vegetable except potatoes with fish, and rarely those. The vegetable follows as a separate course, even when the fish is the main dish of the meal.

CHAPTER IX

OUT OF THE FRYING PAN

A CLATTER and a yell from the kitchen! I dropped my book and raced down the long flagged passage, meeting, as I went, a dense cloud of stifling, stinking smoke, which poured out of the kitchen door. The wails grew louder and more heartrending at each instant.

"Colette!" cried I. "Whatever on earth is the matter?"

"Oh, oh!" sobbed Colette, through the folds of the apron which she had twisted tragically round her head. "*Quel malheur! Ah, mon Dieu, que je suis malheureuse! Jamais, jamais de la vie n'ai-je vu une affaire pareille!* Oh . . . !"

"Colette! Dear, good Colette! Try to tell me — just plainly once — *where* have you burnt yourself?" For the awful smell was certainly one of burning, and I could n't see Colette clearly for the smoke that filled the kitchen.

"Burnt myself?" Colette whisked the apron off her head and rounded on me in a state of furious astonishment. "As if I would cry because I had only burnt *myself!* I've *burnt the friture!*"

I had been horribly frightened, for I love Colette. The relief of her explanation, joined to its absurdity, were too much for me. I sat down and crowed — literally crowed with hysterical laughter — till Colette, growing frightened

Out of the Frying Pan

in her turn, opened the window and forced a drink of water on me. Then, when we were both quiet and reasonable again, she turned reproachful.

"It is nothing to laugh at, you know. The *friture* costs so dear, and it ought to last for months and months. No, indeed, it is no laughing matter! It is on my conscience that I have been negligent — but, figure to yourself, I do but turn my back a little, little moment — the fire is very quick — I smell something — I throw myself upon the *friture* — but it is too late. *Ah! Mon Dieu! Quel malheur!*"

"Don't start that noise again. I'll buy you some more to-morrow."

"But I think of the waste. In these hard days —"

"How much does it cost?" (*Friture*, I may as well explain, means a big pan of dripping, in which things are fried.)

"To make a good, big *friture*, in my large, deep pan — oh, one has for fifteen francs' worth of fat. But I will not ask for all that — I will try to manage with the half quantity. I am so sorry — so ashamed —"

"You needn't be. Tell me all the things you mean to cook in the *friture*, and I will make an article for the cook book. So you will help me to earn the fifteen francs and perhaps even a little more to put in my pocket. You see, there is no need to be sorry or ashamed, *mon amie*. It is a good turn that you do me — not a bad one at all."

Colette was silent for a moment. Then she said, in an unusually gentle little voice.

"*Merci, ma petite — merci beaucoup!*" And I knew that she meant it very much indeed, or she would never have forgotten her carefully acquired manners enough to call me "*petite*", as if I were twelve years old again, and home from my convent for the holidays.

Colette's Best Recipes

Before telling about the dishes cooked in the *friture* (which is Colette's name for the big pan of dripping in which things are fried) it may be well to say a word, first of all, as to the *friture* itself. Any kind of nice dripping will do, provided that it is rendered down and cleansed — not clarified, but just cleansed — by having cut away from it any dark matter that may fall to the bottom when the dripping is set. It should be kept in the pan in which it is used, this pan being deep and large enough to take in the frying basket easily. Before each using, warm the pan just a tiny trifle, to loosen the hard cake of dripping from the sides. Slip it out, turn it upside down, and scrape away any little burnt bits that you may find at the bottom. By this means, the fat is kept always clean and nice.

Colette does not use a real frying pan for her deep frying. She has a round iron pan, about twelve inches deep, with a little round handle at each side. An ordinary frying pan is not good for *friture* work; it is only good for sautéed things and for omelettes.

Colette always keeps two sets of *friture*, — the big one for things in general, and the little one for fish. You can do fish in the general *friture*, if you like, but you always run the risk of tanging the fat, with the result that you will get fishy fritters and sweets for the rest of the chapter.

There is nothing equal to good beef dripping for the *friture*. There is nothing equal to fresh butter for eggs and omelettes, cooked in an open frying pan; lard makes a good second.

Oil fries things to a most lovely color and makes them very crisp, but it is more costly than fat and not quite so easy to use.

Margarine should never be used for frying under any circumstances whatever.

Out of the Frying Pan

1. FRITURE BATTER. Put into a good-sized basin half a pound flour, one tablespoonful of brandy, one tablespoonful of olive oil, and a pinch of salt (no salt if the batter is for a sweet dish). The best way of arranging matters is to sift the salt into the flour, and then make a hole in the center and pour in the oil and brandy. Pour in also a little cold water, and begin to mix from the center, stirring all the time with a wooden spoon. When you have put in enough water to make a mixture of the consistency of whipped cream, begin to beat across and across, raising the spoon well at each stroke, so that plenty of air may get into the batter. When you have beaten for five minutes, put the batter aside and let it stand in a cool place for two hours.

It is not possible to tell the exact quantity of water that you will want, because the amount differs with different kinds of flour. But the batter should be thick enough to coat the back of a metal spoon: also it ought to follow the spoon in a kind of thread, which breaks, of course, when it is an inch or two long. On the other hand, it must not be thick enough to make lumps; it must be a running mixture, not a paste.

2. FLEMISH BATTER is very cheap and convenient, and many people like it better than the French kind, as it is lighter and crisper. Remember that it must be used as soon as ever it is made, so get the fat heated beforehand and prepare all that is wanted, in order that you may waste no time.

Sift together in a basin half a pound of flour, one teaspoonful sugar, and one teaspoonful baking powder. Add a little beer or soda water, to mix the whole to the consistency of an ordinary frying batter, and use immediately.

Colette seldom makes batter with an egg. She says it

Colette's Best Recipes

is wasteful. But, if she has a white left over from something else, she often uses it in the following way for a

3. SWEET BATTER.

    ½ pound flour
    1 teaspoonful sugar
    A pinch of salt
    Sweet milk to mix
    The white of the egg, whipped to the stiffest possible froth

Mix it like number one, adding the whipped white of the egg at the last moment.

CERVELLE FRITE (FRIED OX BRAINS). A delicious lunch dish or entrée. Clean the brains carefully, and soak them for one hour in cold salt and water to take out the blood. Put them into a pan with enough cold water to cover them, with pepper, salt, half a lemon sliced, and three small onions. Cover the pan and boil gently till tender. Drain the brains. Cut them into pieces the size of an egg. Dip them in the *friture* batter.

Now heat the *friture* till it stops bubbling, and begins to give off a thin blue smoke. Try it with a bit of bread. If the bread turns crisp and brown at once, the *friture* is ready. Put in the pieces of brains, one at a time, with a little pause between each. Leave plenty of room in the pan, so that they may not touch each other. Fry them to a good golden brown. Take them out with a drainer, and put them on a sieve with a plate underneath, so that whatever fat too much there may be will drip through the sieve on to the plate, from which it may be scraped off and used again. Keep them very hot. Pile them on a hot dish and garnish with parsley before serving.

Any other kind of brains may be served in the same way, though most others — calf's brains, for instance — need only a few moments of boiling before they are fried.

Out of the Frying Pan

CROQUETTES DE VEAU (CROQUETTES OF VEAL). Another delightful dish for lunch, supper, or breakfast. You may prepare any kind of white meat in the same way, — chicken, rabbit, or pork.

Melt in a pan two tablespoonfuls of lard or butter. Add one tablespoonful of chopped parsley, pepper, salt, a grate of nutmeg, and two tablespoonfuls of flour, well piled up. Stir all together with a wooden spoon, and when well mixed over the fire, add slowly a small cupful of hot milk, or, if you prefer, a little good gravy. Stir the sauce over the fire till it becomes as thick as porridge. Cut your meat into very neat little squares — quite tiny, please — and mix them into the sauce. It is best not to mince the meat through a machine, because it loses its character if you do so. Let the mixture get quite cold, and then you will find it firm enough to handle. Shape it into small croquettes and roll them in fine white crumbs. Beat up an egg. Dip the croquettes into it. Crumb them again. Drop them into deep fat, heated to smoking point, and cook them just like the brains. Serve them very hot indeed, garnished with fried parsley.

When they are cut, their crisp brown outsides are found to hide a sort of creamy filling, with little bits of meat in it. Delicious!

PETITES PÂTES, FRITES (LITTLE FRIED PIES). Take one pound of any nice short pastry that you know best how to make. Roll it out to the thickness of quarter of an inch and cut it into circles with something just a trifle larger than a tumbler. Dampen the edges of the circles. Now mince any cooked meat that you happen to have, season it well with pepper, salt, mixed spice, and, if you like, a little grated onions or chopped parsley. Add to it enough good gravy to make a rather damp paste of it. Put a large spoonful on one side of a round of pastry, double the other side over, press the edges together, and pinch them up and down with your fingers, to make a sort of frilly border. Now, you have things the shape of English turnovers. Drop them into the *friture*, which has been heated to smoking point, and fry them a nice bright brown. Keep them very hot indeed till the moment of service comes. Pile them up in a folded napkin when they go to table.

If nicely fried, they will be as dry and crisp as if they had been baked. This is a very economical method of using up leavings of cold meat. Cold fish can also be employed in the same way, while a spoonful of jam folded into the pastry gives a sort of little sweet pie very dear to the hearts of children. Colette always used to make them for me, with strawberry jam inside, when I came home for the holidays. She used to roll them in sifted sugar as soon as they came out of the pan, I remember, to make them more fascinating still.

BEIGNETS D'HUITRES (FRITTERED OYSTERS). Take the oysters from their shells and drop them into boiling water to which the juice of a lemon has been added. Let them cook in it for half an hour. Drain them thoroughly. Sprinkle them generously with pepper and salt. Dip them into the *friture* batter and fry them in deep fat heated to smoking point. Pile them up high in a dish, and garnish them with fried parsley. This is a delicious entrée or lunch dish. It would also be good at supper.

BOULETTES (RISSOLES OF COLD MEAT). Mince one pound of any sort of cold meat, with quarter of a pound of cooked bacon, — rather fat, if possible, unless the meat happens to be fat also. Now boil two pounds of potatoes, drain them very dry, and put them through a potato press. Mix well into the meat, adding pepper, salt, and a tiny bit of grated onion or garlic. Now beat up two eggs very well. Mix them into the other ingredients and roll all into wee balls, — the smaller the prettier. Dip them in flour, brush them over lightly with beaten egg, and roll them in fine white crumbs. Put them in the frying basket and plunge them into deep fat heated to smoking point. Let them get well colored. Drain thoroughly. They swell little in cooking and become very light and good. Make a thick tomato sauce — see article on sauces — pile up the Boulettes in a high pyramid at the middle of a hot dish, and pour tomato sauce round the base of it. Serve at once.

BŒUF À L'HUILE (COLD BEEF FRIED IN OIL). Cut cold boiled beef into thin, neat slices. Rub each slice well with a bead of cut garlic. Put into an open frying pan enough oil just to cover the bottom. Heat it till it smokes. Put in as many slices of beef as will lie flat at the bottom of the pan and fry them lightly at both sides. Sprinkle them well with pepper and salt. When all the slices are fried, arrange them on a hot dish, heat two tablespoonfuls of vinegar in the pan and pour it over all. Serve at once.

BEIGNETS DE VOLAILLE (GAME FRITTERS). Take the breast only of a game bird of any kind, roasted and cold, and divide each side of it into four or six long and rather thin pieces. Soak the pieces in vinegar for half an hour. Drain them very dry. Dust them with pepper and salt. Dip them into *friture* batter, and fry in the usual way.

Prepare chicken in the same way. If the dish is for family use, you may also cut up the other parts of the bird, taking the fleshy pieces from the legs, and making big, fat fritters of them.

BEIGNETS DE CHOUX FLEURS (CAULIFLOWER FRITTERS). Take the flowers only and break them into neat little sprays. Wash them very well and boil them in salt and water till they are tender. Drain them. Sprinkle them with salt, pepper, and a few drops of vinegar. Dip them into Flemish batter and fry them in deep fat to smoking point. This is a very pretty and dainty vegetable.

BEIGNETS OF SALSIFY, CHICORY, OR CELERY. Scrape the vegetable, cut it into little pieces about half the size of your least finger, and boil them in salt and water till they are quite tender. Drain them well. Measure the quantity. Make the same amount of well-seasoned white sauce, *very thick*. Mix in the vegetables, and spread the whole thing on a dish to get cool. When it is quite cold, it will be so firm that you can cut it into neat little pieces; dip them in Batter No. 1, and fry them in deep fat.

These, like the Croquettes, liquefy as they get hot, and come running out in a delicious cream when the shell is cut.

BEIGNETS DE POMMES DE TERRE (POTATO FRITTERS). Steam your potatoes, peel them while hot, and beat them through a sieve. Add sugar and a very little salt, if you want to make a sweet dish of them; add a good deal of salt and only the merest pinch of sugar, if you want to make a vegetable of them. Mix in enough flour to bind them into a firm, smooth paste. The paste must be well bound, but not so stiff that it is tough. Work it into a ball, roll it out on a floured board to the thickness of half an inch, and cut it into rounds with the edge of a tumbler. Heat your *friture* till it smokes, drop in the rounds, one at a time, and fry them fast. Take them up with a skimmer as soon as they are brown. Let them drip dry, roll them in sifted sugar or sprinkle them with salt, and serve at once. They must be served without a second of delay, for, as soon as they become cold, they fall, and are no longer either pretty or good.

Out of the Frying Pan

If served very hot, with a nice jam or wine sauce, they are the most delicious of puddings.

If served very hot, with a little grilled bacon or ham, they are a breakfast for the gods.

Hand a thick cheese sauce with them, and you have a nice simple savory or supper dish.

CRÊPES (PANCAKES). We eat them here on Shrove Tuesday almost as a matter of religion, and at many other seasons of the year as a matter of pleasure. They are not a bit like the pancakes I have sometimes tasted in England, but much thinner and lighter.

Put into a deep dish one pound of flour. Make a hole at the middle and break three eggs into this hole. Add two tablespoonfuls of brandy, a good pinch of salt, and a tablespoonful of olive oil. By way of flavoring you may add either a little orange-flower water, or the grated rind of a lemon. Add a little cold water and begin to stir from the center with a wooden spoon, putting in water, a few drops at a time, till the mixture is like a thin custard. It should just coat the back of a spoon smoothly but not thickly. Put the dish in a cool place when the batter has been well beaten and leave it for three hours.

Now melt in a small omelette pan a little piece of lard. Pour off into a cup as much of the lard as will come, leaving only enough to grease the bottom of the pan. Put the pan on a brisk heat till it is quite hot, and then, with a tablespoon, pour in the batter, tipping the pan as you do so, in order that the batter may run fast all over the bottom of it. The pan should be entirely covered with the thinnest possible coating of batter.

"It's not easy to do the first time," said Colette. "You want the trick of it. The first time one does it, one cannot tip fast enough, and the *crêpe* turns into a thick dab, in-

Colette's Best Recipes

stead of into the lightest and daintiest of thin skins at the bottom of the pan. However, it soon comes."

Let the *crêpe* fry for a moment, and, when it is brown underneath, turn it and fry the other side, too.

"They can tell if it is brown underneath by lifting up a corner and looking underneath," Colette explains. "The right way to turn it is to give the handle of the pan a sharp tap, and then the *crêpe* jumps."

"Yes. Up into one's face. One needs to wear a mask when making *crêpes*," said I ruefully.

"La, la! Every one is not as clumsy as you! Tell them they can turn it with two knives if they like better. When it is fried on the second side, slip it off on to a hot plate, and keep it in an oven which is just cool enough not to dry it, but plenty warm enough not to let it go limp, while you are doing the others."

When all are done, fold them, pile them up in a scaffolding on a dish, sprinkle them with lots of sifted sugar, and garnish them with slices of cut lemon.

The batter must be constantly stirred all the time the frying is going on, so that the thick part may not drop down to the bottom.

CRÊPES AUX POMMES (APPLE PANCAKES). Make the batter as above. Take very nice cooking apples, of a kind that easily softens in heat. Peel them. Take out the cores with a corer. Cut them into wafer-thin slices, going right across the apple at each slice. Just before frying the *crêpes*, stir the apples into the batter, and, when frying, try to arrange things so that at least two good slices are in each *crêpe*.

Don't fold them — you can't, without spoiling the pieces of apple. Lay them flat on a hot dish, sprinkling each thickly with powdered sugar.

Out of the Frying Pan

BÂTONETTES (FRIED STICKS). Make a store of these at a time and keep them to serve with stewed fruits, custards, and other soft sweets of the same kind. They can be stored in a tin and reheated in the oven when wanted. They are excellent, and they give a novel look to any very simple and everyday kind of dessert.

Sift one pound of flour on to the pastry-board, mixing in with it a good teaspoonful of powdered cinnamon and half a pound of sifted sugar. Chop roughly in it half a pound of good butter, and then rub the butter in with the tips of your fingers, till the mixture is like bread crumbs. Make a hole at the center of the flour. Break an egg into the hole, and add two or three tablespoonfuls of cold water. Begin to mix with your fingers, adding a little more water from time to time, till the whole is of the stiffness of pastry. Knead it just like bread till it leaves your hands quite clean. Then roll it out to the thickness of quarter of an inch, cut it into narrow strips, and twist them, just like cheese straws. Some people turn the strips into little rings; others tie them in wee bows. The paste is so firm and at the same time so flexible that it is easy to handle, and all kinds of pretty things can be made with it. Heat the *friture* to smoking point. Put a few at a time of your dainty things into the frying basket, and lower them in. They will turn bright brown very soon. Shake them quite dry in the basket.

They are crisp and delicious, and, if well fried, so dry that they do not soil your hands in the least when you touch them. They are dry enough to be eaten cold, if necessary; but, like all fried things, they gain by being heated.

PAIN PERDU (BREAD FRITTERS). "I expect they'll know that already, Colette," said I. "It's rather a renowned sort of thing. But, as you make it so deliciously, just tell them your method. Perhaps you may do some little trick or other which is a novelty to them."

Cut slices of bread about half an inch thick. Take away the crusts and make the white into neat squares. Warm one pint of milk till it is about blood heat. Add to it plenty of sugar and a few drops of any flavoring essence that you like best. Put the slices of bread in a single layer in a deep dish and pour the milk over them. There should be enough milk to soak them all well but not enough to float them. Let them soak for one hour. Beat up three eggs with a tiny pinch of salt and three tablespoonfuls of milk, just as if you were going to make an omelette. Put into a large, open frying pan one good tablespoonful of butter. When it is hot, dip into the eggs as many slices of bread as will lie flat in the pan, take them out of the egg with a drainer, and slip them into the hot fat. Let them fry to a good golden brown. Melt another spoonful of butter before turning them to the other side. When they are very well browned on both sides, sprinkle with sifted sugar and serve.

Some people pile a spoonful of strawberry jam on each slice. About the best thing I ever had to eat in England was a pudding called "Beggars on Horseback", which was nothing more or less than Pain Perdu, with hot strawberry jam on it.

But Colette won't put jam. You never met such a pig-headed old piece of obstinacy in your life!

"It is not necessary," says she. "You only want it because you are greedy — but greedy, mon Dieu! Who disgraced herself by eating Pets de Nonne in the open streets of Paris?"

PETS DE NONNE (FRITTER PUFFS) is the very vulgar name of the things that polite folks call BEIGNETS SOUFFLÉS.

Out of the Frying Pan

At the corner of a street in Paris, not far from the Louvre, there is a man with a stall, who fries *Pets de Nonne* and sells them, all crisp and crackling, at a few sous the handful. They are all that there is of the most delicious! But I was a fool to tell Colette that I had succumbed to their charms. She was honestly shocked, and has never got over it. Let me just tell you how to make them.

Put into a pan half a pint of water, one tablespoonful butter, the thinly peeled rind of a lemon, and one tablespoonful sugar. Boil for five minutes, and then take out the lemon. Take a handful of flour in your left hand, hold a wooden spoon in your right, and sprinkle flour into the pan, stirring all the while, till you get a paste so thick that you have difficulty in moving the spoon in it. Keep on boiling and stirring till the mixture leaves the sides of the pan. The more it can be cooked, the nicer it will be, for very well-done flour has a much more delicate flavor than that which is only partly done: but you must never stop stirring, even for a second, or it will burn.

Take the pan off the fire, break in an egg, and beat it till it is most thoroughly mixed into the paste. Then add another, and so on up to four. The more thoroughly the eggs are beaten in, the lighter the Beignets will be.

Have ready your deep pan of fat, heated to smoking point. Take up with the handle of a spoon a little bit of paste no bigger than a walnut. It will puff to the size of an egg, or even bigger, become quite empty, and swim up to the top of the pan. As soon as it is bright brown, fish it out with a drainer, and put in another. Only do one at a time, please. And keep them very hot till they are wanted. Sprinkle them with sugar before serving. No sauce is ever handed with them, but, now and then, a few drops of some strong perfume — lemon, for instance —

Colette's Best Recipes

may be rubbed into the sugar with which they are sprinkled.

If you want to do good deep-pan frying, *always*

1. See that there is a sufficient depth of fat to cover the things that must be fried.

2. See that the fat is heated to smoking point.

3. Put in each bit separately, with a little pause between each pair, so that the fat may reheat again.

4. Keep them as small as possible, so that they may have a chance to get well cooked through.

5. Serve them very hot.

6. Make no extra ones. Fried things don't reheat well.

CHAPTER X

COLETTE COOKS VEGETABLES

IN the North of France, where we live, potatoes are by no means the universal food that they are in England. We eat them, perhaps, three or four times a week: and, when we do have them, they are deliciously cooked. But, especially in the poorer families, the place of honor is taken by dried beans, called Haricots Blancs or Haricots Rouges, according to their color.

They are easier to grow than potatoes and less subject to blight; they can be stored in less space; and a moderate help of them "fills you up" more than the same amount of potato would do, and is, I believe, equally good for you. So they appeal very strongly to a practical-minded person like Colette.

"But the potatoes are more distinguished," she assures me earnestly. "One does not give dried beans except quite in the family. I will tell you about the potatoes first."

So we make a "distinguished" start!

Colette practically always boils her potatoes in their skins, and peels them afterwards. By this means, she gets not only the full flavor, but also the full nourishment, most of which lies just under the skin. The only exceptions that she makes are in favor of very old or very new potatoes. The very new ones get their skins rubbed off, of course, while the very old ones are peeled, so that the bad parts may be cut away.

PURÉE DE POMMES DE TERRE (MASHED POTATOES). This is a very important French dish, — a sort of test case for the cook. If she can't make a good purée, she's no use, however many other qualifications she may have.

Boil and peel the potatoes, and put them through a sieve or a potato press. Pour about half a teacupful of milk into a pan and make it very hot. Stir in the potato, with salt and pepper to taste, and as much butter as you can spare. A dish of purée for four people should have a piece of butter at least the size of an egg, and as much more as you care to add. Put the pan on a moderate heat, and stir the purée with a wooden spoon, adding more milk as required, till it is thinned down to exactly the consistency of whipped cream. Then draw the pan aside, and let it simmer gently, giving it a stir now and then, till it is very hot indeed all through. Pour into a heated dish, smooth the surface with a knife, and serve at once.

Mistakes folks make with purée.

1. They get it too thick. It must not be thicker than cream unless it is going to be made up afterwards into something else, — *boulettes*, for example.

2. They don't heat it all through. It takes a long while to get well heated up, — at least fifteen minutes.

3. They try to heat it too fast, and it scorches; it's a terror to scorch, and quite uneatable when once the accident has happened.

4. They make it with cold potatoes instead of with fresh-boiled ones, and then it is sticky and heavy and horribly indigestible.

The only good way to reheat cold purée is to smooth it into a pie dish or *au gratin* dish, put little bits of butter

Colette Cooks Vegetables

here and there on top, and bake it in a brisk oven to a good brown. Sometimes Colette does the fresh purée like this and calls it Gâteau de Pommes de Terre. But it isn't really. This is the real thing:

GÂTEAU DE POMMES DE TERRE (POTATO CAKE). Make three cupfuls of purée, rather stiffer than usual. Beat in the yolks of two eggs. Whip the whites to the stiffest possible froth, fold them into the mixture, put all into a buttered dish, which must not be more than three-quarters full, and bake in a brisk oven till the Gâteau is well risen and browned. Serve it quickly, in the dish in which it was cooked.

VARIATIONS. 1. Add three heaped tablespoonfuls of grated cheese, a little extra pepper, and a little mustard. Fill small ramekin cases. Sprinkle the tops with grated cheese and brown well. This makes a nice little supper dish or savory.

2. Spread a layer of minced and well-seasoned meat or fish under the potato. In this case, one egg will be enough; two would make the dish too rich.

3. Add a little sugar and lemon peel, reduce the salt almost to nothing, and you have a nice, simple pudding.

POMMES DE TERRE DORÉES (GILDED POTATOES). Take small potatoes — new ones are best — peel them, and cut them all, as nearly as possible, to the same size. Fry them in an open frying pan, till they are a pretty gold color all over. Put them into a saucepan, with just one teacupful of water, and let them cook gently till they are quite tender. The pan should remain covered and should be shaken from time to time. Drain them out carefully. Potatoes cooked in this way are not at all unlike potatoes roasted under the joint, but rather softer.

POMMES DE TERRE SAUTÉES (TOSSED POTATOES). Boil

Colette's Best Recipes

the potatoes in their skins till they are quite done but not broken at all. Peel them while they are hot. Melt in an open frying pan enough good dripping or lard to cover the bottom well. Cut the potatoes into slices about quarter of an inch thick and fry them, tossing them now and then till they are a good golden brown. Sprinkle with salt and serve very hot.

Cold potatoes, sliced and sautéed, are quite eatable; but they never taste like fresh ones, and never will, so don't waste your hopes on them.

POMMES DE TERRE SOUFFLÉES (PUFFED POTATOES). Peel the raw potatoes and cut them into rounds the thickness of a cracker biscuit.

Have two pans of deep fat on the fire. Let one be just melted, and the other so very hot that it has stopped bubbling and has begun to give off a thin blue smoke.

Put the potatoes first into the pan of just melted fat. As soon as they begin to color, fish them out with a drainer, let them drip a moment, and then toss them into the very hot fat. You will see that, in a few seconds, they puff up enormously, becoming almost like balls in shape. Fish them out, drain them quickly, keeping them very hot all the while, and serve them promptly, powdered with salt. The right way to serve them is to wrap them in a warm table napkin, so that they may not catch cold and fall flat on their way to the dining room.

Put only a few potatoes at a time in the second pan. If you put too many, they won't puff.

POMMES DE TERRE À LA PARISIENNE (PARIS POTATOES). Put into a saucepan a piece of butter or good dripping the size of an egg. Slice a large onion fine and cook it in the fat till it begins to color. Add ten potatoes, peeled and cut in halves lengthwise, one pint water, pepper, salt, and a

Colette Cooks Vegetables

little bunch of sweet herbs. Let all cook gently, like a stew, till the potatoes are tender. Drain them out, put them in a hot dish, and strain a little of their liquor around and over them. Any liquor that remains is excellent for soup.

Some people think olive oil nicer for this dish than either butter or dripping.

POMMES DE TERRE À LA SAUCE BLANCHE. Boil the potatoes in their skins, peel them while still very hot, and toss them in a good Sauce Blanche (see page 132).

POMMES DE TERRE À LA MAÎTRE D'HÔTEL. Boil the potatoes in their skins, peel them while still very hot and slice them. Put them in a hot dish, and add Maître d'Hôtel Sauce (see page 133) or Maître d'Hôtel Butter (see page 133).

POMMES DE TERRE EN GALETTES (LITTLE POTATO CAKES). After boiling the potatoes in their skins, put them through a potato press or sieve. Add a piece of butter the size of an egg for each dozen potatoes, salt, pepper, and as much flour as will make the whole stick into a paste, — the less the better. Work all well with your hands till the paste is firm and smooth. Then clean your fingers, dip them in flour, and use them to form small flat cakes. Fry these cakes in lard or olive oil, first on one side and then on the other, using an open frying pan. Serve them very hot, garnished with parsley.

BOULETTES DE POMMES DE TERRE (POTATO BALLS). Make a very thick purée from twelve potatoes. Beat into it pepper, salt, and the yolk of an egg. Let it stand in a cool place all night. Next day form wee balls — certainly not larger than walnuts — brush them over with the beaten white of the egg, roll them in fine white crumbs. Drop them into deep fat which is heated to smoking point. They will puff a good deal and will swim to the surface, turning bright gold in color. Fish them out, drain them, and serve them very hot, piled on a heated napkin.

Colette wishes she knew exactly what sort of dried beans you get in America. But I tell her it really does n't matter, for all beans come to pretty much the same in the end, the only difference being that some take a little longer to cook than others.

All dried vegetables should be washed very well indeed before used; then soaked in cold water overnight; and then cooked in the water in which they were soaked. If you throw away the soaking water, you loose a good deal of the flavor and nourishment of the vegetables with it.

Dried beans should be very well cooked, — so well that you can crush one between your finger and thumb without the least effort. If you are late with them, and you want to hurry them up, stir in a teaspoonful of baking soda. When the effervescence goes down, you will see that the beans are all split and coming out of their skins. In a very few minutes more, they will be done. But this way of going to work is a little extravagant, as it makes the bean water unfit for use in soup afterwards.

HARICOTS À LA BRETONNE (HARICOTS OF BRITTANY). Soak, boil, and drain one pint of beans (measured when dry). Put into an open frying pan a piece of butter — or good beef dripping — the size of an egg. Cut a large onion into fine strips and cook it in the fat till it is pale brown. Add a teaspoonful of flour, and let that brown also. Then add enough of the haricot water to thin out the whole to a little sauce, stir in the haricots, season them well with salt and pepper, and let them warm gently for quarter of an hour.

There should be very little sauce, — only enough to

Colette Cooks Vegetables

soften the beans and stick them together. If there is so much that they can swim in it, the dish will not be right.

HARICOTS DU NORD (NORTHERN HARICOTS). This is the great family dish of the North of France. In houses where there are children, it never fails to appear each time there is a roast.

Boil the beans till they are within quarter of an hour of being done. Drain them. Keep your joint in a good oven till it is nicely browned. Then take it out for a moment, make a good bed of the cooked haricots in the baking tin, lay the joint on them, and finish it like this. Serve them around the meat.

The dripping and the meat juices go into the beans and make them perfectly delicious. They crisp a little if there is a good deal of fat and may even brown. They are very nourishing and extremely nice.

HARICOTS EN PURÉE (MASHED HARICOTS). Do them just like potato purée, but use, if possible, more butter and less milk. Colette often puts a small amount of mashed potato in with the beans, and I consider it a great improvement, as it smooths them down so nicely.

Haricot Beans are also served:

À la Sauce Blanche
À la Sauce Tomate (see chapter on Sauces)
À la Maître d'Hôtel
À la Mayonnaise Verte

"Tell me, Colette, how it is that, when I go to stay in England, the greens taste of nothing but water, while your greens have all sorts of delicious little flavors."

"Because the English drown their vegetables instead of cooking them. *Tiens!* I will give you a few standard French ways of doing things."

CHOUX À LA FRANÇAISE (FRENCH SPICED CABBAGE). Wash the cabbage and boil it in the usual way, in plenty of salt and water. Drain it. Chop it well in the colander, or, if you prefer, put it through the food chopper. Measure it and return it to the pan. To each cupful of cabbage add a level saltspoonful of mixed spice, a level dessertspoonful of butter, and a level teaspoonful of flour. Stir over the fire till the mixture has boiled for three minutes. Then taste it and add salt as required, with the tiniest possible pinch of pepper.

If the butter is salted, you will probably need no more salt. Go lightly on the pepper, as the spice has already a slightly heating taste.

You will find that the flavor of the cabbage comes out to the full, and that it has nothing of that "greens-water" taste, which so many people dislike.

"There are those who don't care for spice," explains Colette, "and, for them, I should use a good pinch of grated nutmeg — about as much as would lie on my thumb-nail to each cupful of cabbage."

CHOUX À LA CRÈME (CREAMED CABBAGE). Choose a cabbage with a nice, firm heart. Remove the outer leaves, cut the heart into four parts, and boil it in salt and water till it is quite tender. Drain it well, and even squeeze out the water, keeping it very hot all the while. Put it in a warmed dish, and cover it with a good Sauce Blanche (see page 131).

CHOUX À LA FLAMANDE (FLEMISH CABBAGE). Boil and drain the cabbage in the usual way, squeeze it well, and chop it roughly. To each cupful of cabbage allow one large onion and a piece of dripping the size of an egg. Melt the dripping in an open pan, add the sliced onion and the cabbage, and fry all till you see that the bits of onion are be-

Colette Cooks Vegetables

ginning to turn brown. Then sprinkle liberally with salt and pepper and serve.

Slices of cold potato are sometimes mixed into the cabbage, but this is not real French cooking at all, it is pure British, though whether Scotch or English is more than I can tell you.

CHOUX ROUGES AUX POMMES (RED CABBAGE WITH APPLES). This is not French either; it is a Dutch recipe, which has wandered over the border into the North of France.

Wash and prepare a red cabbage and put it into a pan with water enough to cover it. Add five apples, peeled and cored, a piece of butter the size of an egg, pepper, salt, and six cloves. Let the whole thing boil two and a half hours on a moderate heat.

Take out the cabbage and dish it, draining it first. Remove the cloves. Stir together one tablespoonful of vinegar, one tablespoonful of currant jelly, and one teaspoonful of corn flour. Stir all this into the sauce and, when it thickens, pour it over the cabbage.

PETITS CHOUX (SPROUTS AND SPRING GREENS). Prepare them and boil them in the usual way in salt and water. Drain them very well. Leave the sprouts whole, but mash greens through the colander, or chop them very thoroughly with a knife.

Cut an onion and rub your frying pan with it, around and around, pressing rather hard, so that you squeeze out a good part of the onion juice into the pan. Then add a large tablespoonful of butter or good dripping, heat it, and toss the greens in it till they are well buttered. Sprinkle them with salt before serving, *not* while they are in the frying pan.

"Why not?"

"Because salt makes the fat fly all about, and then your

stove is spoiled. No one will be able to say that the greens exactly taste of onions; it's such a pity to kill the flavor of the dish by too much seasoning of any kind. But they will know that something or other has been added, which has made the sprouts taste warm and rich, instead of thin and watery."

EPINARDS (SPINACH). French spinach, dandelion greens, and sorrel are never bitter and harsh as they are in other countries. We always boil lettuce with them — one good handful of lettuce to each four handfuls of the other green. The outside leaves of lettuce will do quite well, while the hearts can be kept for salad. The one vegetable softens down the other, and then the addition of a little cream to the purée finishes the business. If you can't get cream, stir up a dessertspoonful of fresh butter in a teacupful of warm milk, and the result will be about the same.

CHOUX FLEURS (CAULIFLOWERS). Take the white part only, none of the stalk or green. Break it into neat little sprigs. Cook them in salt and water, boiling not too fast, till they are tender. Drain them and plunge them into cold water to set them. Then reheat them in Sauce Blanche or Sauce Tomate (see chapter on Sauces). Or dip them in batter and fry them (see chapter on Frying). Or let them get cold and dress them with a mayonnaise. Or cover them with Sauce Blanche, sprinkle them thickly with grated cheese, brown the whole in a sharp oven, and call it CHOUX FLEURS AU GRATIN.

PETITS POIS (GREEN PEAS). Shell the peas and wash them. Drain them. Toss them in as much flour as they will pick up. Now melt a good tablespoonful of butter in a stewpan and toss the peas in it till they are nicely greased all over. Then add one teaspoonful of sifted sugar, one teaspoonful of salt, one good head of lettuce, washed out,

Colette Cooks Vegetables

not pulled to pieces, and enough water to come halfway to the peas as they lie in the pan. Cover the pan and simmer gently till the peas are tender, — one to three hours according to their age.

Some folks put mint into peas, but Frenchwomen never think of such a thing. Peas ought to be rather a soft and sweet kind of vegetable, and the mint is too burning for them. The lettuce gives them the fresh taste that they need, without making them bite the tongue. The sugar helps to get the right touch of sweetness, and also to keep them a good color. When you have sugar, you won't put any soda, naturally; it's not needed for the color, and it would spoil the taste.

Don't strain the peas before you serve them, you know; dish them in the sauce that they have made for themselves. It is a sort of green cream, sweet and smooth, and very good indeed.

CARROTS AT THEIR BEST. Lots of people don't like carrots, because they taste "faded." They are vegetables that can't stand alone; they need something to help them out. Colette prepares them in one of two ways.

1. She adds a spoonful of vinegar and a spoonful of sugar to the water in which she boils them. You would expect the two to contradict each other and give a negative effect. But, as a matter of fact, the vinegar just serves to "tang" the carrots out of their faded taste, while the sugar softens down the vinegar and prevents it from being too noticeable.

2. She boils them plainly in salt and water and drains them well. Then she melts a lump of butter or dripping in a frying pan, slices in an onion, and lets it fry to a nice brown. The slices of onion are cut so thickly that they don't go to pieces in the fat, and it is easy to take them out

with a spoon before putting in the carrots and tossing them. It would not do to leave the pieces of onion — that would be too much — it is only just a hint of the flavor that is wanted to help out the carrots.

CAROTTES À LA CRÈME (CREAMED CARROTS). Peel the carrots and cut them into small dice. Melt in a stewpan a piece of butter the size of an egg (for one and a half pounds of carrots) and toss them in it till they are well buttered. Stir in salt, pepper, a heaped tablespoonful of flour, and a level teaspoonful of sugar. Add enough water just to cover the carrots and stew gently till they are tender (one to four hours, according to the time of year). Draw the pan off the fire and stir in enough cream to make the sauce opaque, — the more the better. Turn all into a hot dish and sprinkle with chopped parsley.

CAROTTES À LA FLAMANDE (FLEMISH CARROTS). Peel one pound of carrots and quarter of a pound of onions. Put them through the food chopper together. Toss them in a tablespoonful of flour and a good pinch of salt and pepper. Put them into a stewpan with enough brown gravy or good stock just to cover them and stew gently till they are perfectly tender. Turn all into a hot dish and garnish with wedges of fried bread.

HARICOTS VERTS (FRENCH BEANS). We never cut these beans into little bits, as they do in England. We simply pull out the threads and, if they are very large, break them in half. Then they must be thrown into fast-boiling salt and water, cooked at the gallop till they are tender, drained, and dressed.

The most common dressing — and I think the nicest — consists of merely tossing the beans in a little hot butter or good olive oil, and sprinkling them well with salt and pepper before sending them to table.

Colette Cooks Vegetables

Another very favorite way of serving them is to take some of the dripping from the roast, fry in it a small quantity of chopped onion, and then add the beans, and fry them till they are lightly browned. They must be served very hot indeed.

They are also tossed, sometimes, in a Sauce Blanche, but this is rather rare. When Colette does it I know that her beans are not first class, and that they need the sauce to help them down.

They are very often allowed to get cold and then served in a plain oil and vinegar salad dressing, either alone or with slices of cold potato.

TOMATES EN HORS-D'ŒUVRE. Cut very ripe tomatoes into thin, neat slices and arrange them on round plates, letting the slices overlap each other, like the petals of a daisy. Sprinkle them well with pepper and salt and add to the salt the smallest possible pinch of sugar. Make a plain dressing, two parts of oil to one part of vinegar, pour it over them, cover them with a plate, and let them stand two hours. Sprinkle with chopped parsley and serve.

TOMATES FARCIES (STUFFED TOMATOES). Take six large tomatoes. Cut a little hole the size of a sixpence at the top of each and scoop out about a dessertspoonful of the pulp.

Heat two tablespoonfuls of olive oil in a small pan. Add half a bead of garlic, finely chopped, salt, pepper, a little powdered mushroom if you have any, and sufficient crumbs of white bread to make a thick stuffing.

Fill the tomatoes, letting a little of the stuffing stand up on top of each. Pour one tablespoonful of olive oil into a fireproof dish, stand up the tomatoes in it, and bake them in a brisk oven, basting them often. When they are quite tender, sprinkle each with a wee pinch of chopped parsley, before sending them to table.

Colette's Best Recipes

TOMATES AU GRATIN (TOMATOES WITH CHEESE). Cut a bead of garlic and rub a fireproof dish with it. Then butter the dish liberally and sprinkle it with a good bed of crumbs and grated cheese, mixed together. Arrange on it very ripe tomatoes, which are all about the same size. Put on each a pile of grated cheese and crown the cheese with a lump of butter. Sprinkle all with salt and red pepper. Cook in an oven hot enough to brown the cheese well.

CHAMPIGNONS (MUSHROOMS). If you are doubtful whether your mushrooms are true ones or fungi, here is an infallible test.

Cut a large onion in two and put it to boil in a pan of water with three or four of the doubtful mushrooms. If, at the end of fifteen minutes, the onion remains its natural color, you may be sure that the mushrooms are good: but if it turns even a very little black or gray, you should not venture to eat them.

CROÛTE AUX CHAMPIGNONS (MUSHROOMS ON HORSEBACK). Peel one pound of mushrooms, throwing them, as you peel them, into vinegar and water. Have ready a pan of boiling, salted water, put in the mushrooms, and boil for five minutes. Drain them well.

Make half a pint of nice Sauce Blanche, beat into it the yolk of an egg, and stir on the fire till the egg thickens. (But it must not boil.) After adding the mushrooms take the pan off the fire, let it cool three minutes, and add the juice of a lemon. Let the pan stand at the side of the fire, where it will keep warm without coming anywhere near to boiling.

Take a large slice of bread, nearly an inch thick. Fry it on both sides in butter. Put it on a hot dish and pour the mushrooms over it.

It is convenient for service if you cut the fried bread into several pieces.

Colette Cooks Vegetables

CHAMPIGNONS SAUTÉS AUX FINES HERBES (MUSHROOMS WITH SWEET HERBS). Blanch the mushrooms as above. Drain them well. Put into a pan two tablespoonfuls of the best olive oil; half a bead of garlic, grated; pepper, salt, and chopped parsley. Toss the mushrooms till they are well buttered and serve very hot.

CHAMPIGNONS EN COQUILLES (MUSHROOM SHELLS). Prepare them exactly as for Croûte aux Champignons. Fill scallop shells, sprinkle them with crumbs, and pour a little melted butter over. Brown them in a brisk oven.

CHAMPIGNONS À LA RUSSE (RUSSIAN MUSHROOMS). Peel one pound of mushrooms, cut them in halves, and let them cook gently in a small pan, with a piece of butter the size of an egg, salt, pepper, and a little grated nutmeg. When they are so cooked that they yield to the pressure of your finger, add two large tablespoonfuls of thick white sauce, and one of thick sour cream. Let the whole boil up. Turn it into a hot dish, sprinkle with parsley, and serve.

If you use cream that is not turned, you will get ordinary mushrooms, stewed with a good white sauce. It is the sourness of the cream that gives the characteristic touch to the dish.

ARTICHAUTS (ARTICHOKES). Colette wants you to know that, if you can manage to prick your fingers with the tips of the leaves of an artichoke, you must n't buy that one, — it is hard and old. The whole of it should be quite green and tender. Wash them well, put them, heavy end downwards, into a big pan of boiling salt and water, and let them boil rather fast till, on pulling one of the leaves, you find that it comes away quite easily. Then put them the other way up on a colander, in a nice warm place, and let them drain at least quarter of an hour. Serve then with a good Sauce Blanche, which contains plenty of butter and not too much salt.

Colette's Best Recipes

ASPERGES (ASPARAGUS). Scrape them. Tie them into small bunches, — not more than twelve heads in a bunch. Throw them into a big pan of boiling salt and water and boil steadily, but not too hard, for fifteen to twenty-five minutes. Drain them. Throw just a splash of cold water on them, to set them. Untie the bunches. When serving *asperges*, give plenty of very good white sauce in a separate tureen.

ASPERGES À L'HUILE (ASPARAGUS SALAD). Let them cool till they are tepid, after boiling them as above. Then hand them with a simple salad dressing of oil and vinegar, containing lots of pepper and a little salt.

It would be a grave fault to offer them *quite* cold. When they are perfectly cold, they must either go into the soup, or be served with a mayonnaise dressing, or be chopped small and mixed into scrambled eggs: this last way, I think, is quite an ideal manner of disposing of "left-over" *asperges*.

SALAD SEASONINGS. When you make salad in America, I wonder if you use all the following seasonings? Each one of them is delicious.

1. Rub a dozen mint leaves in your fingers, to bruise them, and then soak them in four tablespoonfuls of vinegar. At the end of an hour, drain off the vinegar and use it for the dressing of an ordinary lettuce salad, with olive oil, salt, pepper, and the tiniest possible touch of sugar. You never tasted a fresher, cleaner salad in your life. It is just the ideal for thirsty weather.

2. Take green, freshly formed seeds of nasturtiums, chop them finely, and use them for sprinkling the surface of a pale-colored salad, on which they will show up well. They have a hot, clean, mustard taste, which is generally much liked.

Colette Cooks Vegetables

3. Do you put a little sugar into your mayonnaise, always? It is so important, and there are some people who forget it. The right amounts are a mustard spoonful each of sugar and mustard to one egg.

4. Do you know what a good plan it is to pick a bunch of mixed herbs — thyme, mint, sage, laurel, and parsley — tie them up in a bit of muslin with two cloves, and simmer them gently in one pint of vinegar for an hour? Keep the lid on the pan. At the end of the hour, strain the vinegar and bottle it for use. When aromatized in this way, it is splendid for salads of any kind.

When you are cooking vegetables, remember:

Potatoes, onions, carrots, and almost all other root vegetables cook very much better and more quickly in soft water than in hard.

If you want potatoes to cook quickly, cut them in halves lengthwise. Cutting them across is no good, but lengthwise cutting reduces the cooking time by about one third.

If you want to cook carrots — or other root vegetables — in a shorter time than usual, add a good lump of dripping to their water.

Put salt in the water with potatoes, even when you are boiling them in their skins. A little of it gets through the skin and helps the flavor of the vegetable.

When you are scraping salsify, Jerusalem artichokes, or any other delicate white things of the same kind, throw them into vinegar and water, to keep them from going black.

If you want to keep greens from boiling over, slip in a little lump of dripping at the edge of the bubbling pan. The fat will spread over the surface and smooth the bubbles right down.

Don't be too generous with baking soda in your greens;

Colette's Best Recipes

it makes them cook all to bits, and a very tiny lump will keep their color good, just as well as a big knob.

Keep the stalks of cabbage and cauliflower and add them to the soup pot. They give ever such a nice flavor.

Keep all your vegetable waters, if they have no soda in them. All, with the exception, perhaps, of cabbage water, are good for flavoring the soup.

CHAPTER XI

COLETTE MAKES SAUCES

"HOW is it that French sauces are always so good?" people often ask.

I think it is partly due to the fact that we have such a great variety of them, to suit so many different dishes. I shall not be able to do more than suggest just a few in this chapter, — a mere nothing in comparison to the multitude that exist. Also, I think, much of the success is due to the care that is taken in the cooking. A French sauce is not just a little trimming, to be tossed together at the last moment; it is a matter of thought and planning and long attention. But most of all, I think, is due to the almost universal use of roux, and it is to the fact that their sauces are often thickened with roux, instead of having flour boiled in them, that French cooks owe the delicate creaminess of their dressings. An ordinary sauce, with the flour just boiled in it, does n't always get cooked sufficiently; unless a good deal of time and patience are spent on it, the chances are that the flour will taste raw, harsh, and poor. The roux are cooked beforehand, so that danger is avoided. I will tell you just how Colette manages them.

A BROWN ROUX for thickening soups, gravies, etc., and for coloring them at the same time, is a most valuable thing. Colette hates browning in bottles, and only uses it now and then, always under protest.

Colette's Best Recipes

If you make roux in this way, it will keep for months. Colette does a big jarful at a time and stores it in the cellar.

Take one pound of butter or the best beef dripping, and melt it in an enameled stewpan. When it is quite melted, strain it, to get out any sediment that may be at the bottom. Now stir in one pound two ounces of the best flour, which should first have been dried and sifted. Put the pan on the fire and keep stirring all the while, with a wooden spoon, till the mixture turns a good brown. Now draw the pan away and keep on stirring till the mixture ceases to fizzle, which it will do for several minutes after the pan has left the fire. Have ready an onion, peeled and cut in halves. Put this into the pan as soon as it leaves the fire, to give a little flavor. When no more sound is to be heard, fish out the onion, pour the roux into a stone or earthenware jar, and leave it to get cold. When set, it is just soft enough to be taken out with a spoon.

Now, suppose that you have a soup or a gravy or anything else of the same kind that wants thickening. All you have to do is to bring your liquid to the boil and then stir in one, two, or more spoonfuls of brown roux. The liquid thickens immediately, is perfectly smooth and free from lumps, and needs no more cooking at all.

The brown roux may also be used for fish and vegetable sauces. A little good potato water, with brown roux stirred into it, and pepper and salt added to taste, makes a very simple but quite presentable sauce for everyday vegetables.

A WHITE ROUX. For cream sauces, sweet sauces, etc., a white roux is necessary. It should, if possible, be made with the best fresh butter, as you know dripping won't go well in sweet sauces. It does not keep quite as long as the brown roux, because it is less thoroughly cooked.

Colette Makes Sauces

Therefore, in our little household, Colette only makes up a half quantity at a time.

She melts half a pound of butter in a pan and stirs in nine ounces of flour. She does it exactly like the brown roux, except that she does not allow it to change color. At the first hint of darkening, the pan must come off the fire at once. No onion, naturally!

When you want to make a cream sauce, or a sweet sauce, all that you have to do is to bring the milk, or fruit juice, or syrup up to the boil and then stir in a little white roux. Here are a few examples of good sauces thickened with roux.

SAUCE ROBERT (POOR MAN'S GRAVY). This is the ideal thing for warming up cold meat. It looks and tastes exactly like fresh gravy a trifle thickened. Use four small onions, four good sprigs of parsley, one bay leaf, pepper and salt, half a teaspoonful made mustard, one tablespoonful vinegar. Put the parsley, bay leaf, and onion to boil in just enough water to cover them. Let them cook for three quarters of an hour. Then strain off the liquid and bring it up to the boil again. Add the seasoning. If you like, thicken the sauce with a teaspoonful of brown roux.

SAUCE TOMATE (TOMATO SAUCE). This is made with six tomatoes, two large shallots, one bay leaf, four good sprigs of parsley, half a cupful cold water, pepper, salt, two tablespoonfuls white roux, one cupful milk.

Put the five first-named ingredients together in a small pan and let them boil rather fast for half an hour. Pass them through a sieve. Reheat the liquid. Smooth the roux in a little cold milk. Bring the rest of the milk to the boil. Add the smoothed roux and the seasoning to the hot tomato mixture; stir with a wooden spoon till it thickens; then thin out the sauce as much as you like with the hot milk.

Eat it with croquettes, with fish, with vegetables that need a taste lent to them, with rice or macaroni or any other cereal of that sort, and, last but not least, heat up slices of cold meat in it and they will be better than a fresh stew.

Sauce Piquante

1 pint meat boilings or fish water
2 chopped shallots
3 tablespoonfuls vinegar
1 tablespoonful chopped pickle
1 tablespoonful chopped parsley

Put the shallot with the vinegar into a pan and boil them till all the vinegar is gone. Its flavor will remain in the shallot, but the actual liquid might spoil the consistency of the sauce, so it must be boiled away. Add the meat boilings, pickle, and parsley, with a good allowance of pepper and a little salt. Boil gently for five minutes. Then thicken with brown roux.

This is a very useful sauce for all kinds of made-up meat dishes.

SAUCE ITALIENNE (ITALIAN SAUCE) is exactly the same, with the addition of a couple of tablespoonfuls of mixed herbs, and a dessertspoonful of currant jelly, which should be stirred in at the last moment.

SAUCE À L'OIGNON (ONION SAUCE). Chop four onions fine and boil them in one pint of water till they are perfectly tender. Thicken with white roux. Add salt, pepper, and the smallest possible pinch each of mace and brown sugar.

Another way of making this sauce is to use only the water in which the onions have been boiled whole.

Almost any vegetable which gives a nice liquor, — celery, salsify, mushrooms, Jerusalem artichokes, etc. — can be served with a sauce made of the liquor thickened with a little brown roux.

Colette Makes Sauces

Any meat that has been boiled or stewed can have a simple sauce made for it from its own liquor, thickened with brown roux, well seasoned with salt, pepper, and a tablespoonful of any bottled essence that you have at hand.

That will give you a working notion of the way to handle roux, won't it? Now we must get on to boiled flour sauces, which have to be used when there is no roux at hand. The foundation of all of them is

SAUCE BLANCHE. Use two cupfuls of milk — or milk and cream, — two level tablespoonfuls of butter or three of margarine, three of flour.

Melt the butter in a clean aluminum or enamel pan — never in an iron pan, for it will change the color of the sauce and give a bad taste also. Stir in the flour with a wooden spoon. In another pan have ready the milk, heated to boiling point. When the flour and fat mixture has cooked till it leaves the sides of the pan — at the end of about two minutes probably — begin to add the boiling milk, a few drops at a time, stirring fast and hard.

This is the critical moment. If you want to avoid lumps you must: 1. Add the milk slowly. 2. Stir constantly till it is all added. 3. Stir always in the same direction. 4. Keep the pan off the fire while adding the first half of the milk, then put it back again while adding the second half.

Keep on stirring till the sauce boils. Then draw the pan to the side of the fire, cover it to prevent a skin from forming, and let the sauce just boil — but only just — for a full fifteen minutes. That's the foundation. Now we come to the different flavorings and colorings, which make the difference between one cream sauce and another.

SAUCE AUX CÂPRES (CAPER SAUCE). Stir one tablespoonful chopped capers into one pint Sauce Blanche. Let it simmer beside the fire quarter of an hour. Taste it. If it is flat and dull, let it cool a little, and then add a few drops of vinegar, with about quarter of a tablespoonful of made mustard smoothed in them, to pick up the taste.

SAUCE VERTE (PARSLEY SAUCE). Add two tablespoonfuls chopped parsley to a Sauce Blanche, after the pan has been taken off the fire.

SAUCE AU BEURRE D'ANCHOIS (ANCHOVY SAUCE). Add one to two tablespoonfuls of pounded anchovies or anchovy essence to one pint of Sauce Blanche. No salt, but lots of pepper.

SAUCE BLANCHE, PIQUANTE. Make one cupful thick white sauce, and let it get quite cold. Stir into it one tablespoonful made mustard and two tablespoonfuls vinegar, with salt and pepper to taste. Use as a mayonnaise. Add the mustard a little at a time, tasting often, so that the flavor may not be too strong.

MAYONNAISE AU BEURRE (BUTTER MAYONNAISE). Make one cupful of good white sauce. While it is still warm, beat into it one large tablespoonful of butter and the juice of a large lemon. Add plenty of pepper and salt. Serve cold. This is finer in taste than the former sauce. It goes excellently with salmon and with boiled fish of all kinds.

SAUCE FROIDE À LA CRÈME (COLD CREAM SAUCE). Make a cupful of good white sauce, not very thick. After boiling it for ten minutes take it off the fire and beat in the yolk of an egg, with pepper and salt to taste. Let it stand ten minutes. Then add two tablespoonfuls of white vinegar. Let it stand again till cold. Then beat up the white of the egg to the stiffest possible froth and fold it in gently. This is a splendid sauce for cold fish or salad of any kind.

Then there is all the large tribe of cold, uncooked sauces,

Colette Makes Sauces

to which real Mayonnaise belongs. In England, they often call them Salad Dressings, though the name is not, strictly speaking, correct at all. They are used on every possible kind of cold thing, as well as, now and then, on hot vegetables and eggs.

SAUCE MAÎTRE D'HÔTEL. Melt two tablespoonfuls butter. Stir into it half a teaspoonful chopped parsley, one teaspoonful white vinegar; salt and pepper to taste. Toss vegetables in it, particularly potatoes, or pour it over eggs or fish.

SAUCE PRINTANIÈRE (SPRING SAUCE). Wash and chop a small bouquet of parsley, celery tops, and cress. Boil two eggs hard and put their yolks through a fine hair sieve with the herbs. Put the pressed mixture into a small bowl and use a wooden spoon to mix into it slowly four tablespoonfuls olive oil, two tablespoonfuls white vinegar, two teaspoonfuls made mustard, pepper, and salt. When all is thoroughly mixed, serve in a sauce boat, and pass with fish of almost any kind. This is easier to make than mayonnaise and quite as nice.

One of the handiest things in the world, and yet a thing that is seldom found outside a French kitchen, is

MAÎTRE D'HÔTEL BUTTER. Put a tablespoonful — or more, according to the amount needed — of butter into a saucer; use a small wooden spoon to work into it pepper, salt, a little very finely chopped parsley, and just one drop of citric acid to each tablespoonful of butter. When it is well mixed, work it into a little cake, and lay this cake on the boiled potatoes, peas, or other vegetables; on a chop or steak and then you won't want any gravy; or roll it into pea-sized balls, and dot a dish of cold fish or salad with them.

It should be allowed to melt, if it is served on anything

Colette's Best Recipes

hot. It takes the place of any other sauce or gravy, and is always good and always handy.

REAL MAYONNAISE is a thing which may be made in as many different ways as coffee: and, of course, each cook swears by her own method and is prepared to defend it to the death. Colette's way is *very* good indeed, but, in giving it, I do not mean to court your displeasure by holding it up as being better than your own, you know.

Put the yolk only of an egg into a small basin. If the egg can be very fresh — even hot from the nest — so much the better. Take a small wooden spoon and stir with it, going always in the same direction, and dropping olive oil on to the egg, drop by drop, till you have added three teaspoonfuls. If the mixture becomes very thin, stop dropping and stir only. Add a grain of pepper, two grains of salt, one grain of sugar, and half a teaspoonful of vinegar, quarter of a teaspoonful made mustard.

Add three more teaspoonfuls of oil, stirring in the same way all the time. Then the vinegar and seasoning again.

Continue in this way up to twelve teaspoonfuls of oil, if the egg will carry so much. The mixture must never be thinner than butter on a hot day. Whenever it thins down, that is a sign that you must do a lot more stirring before adding anything more.

I have been told by another cook, for whom I have a great respect, that it is not good to add the seasonings from time to time, — that you should stir into the yolk of the egg, right at the start, one fourth teaspoonful mustard, one fourth teaspoonful fine sugar, one half teaspoonful salt, a good pinch of red pepper. And add nothing but the oil and vinegar as you go along.

MAYONNAISE VERTE (GREEN MAYONNAISE) is made by adding three tablespoonfuls of mixed and chopped parsley,

Colette Makes Sauces

mint, cress, and the green of baby onions, after the sauce is made.

RÉMOULADE is a very highly-savored sauce, much in vogue for dishes of cold meat. After the plain mayonnaise is made, add to it

> 1 tablespoonful of chopped capers
> 1 tablespoonful chopped pickled onions
> 2 chopped anchovies
> 1 tablespoonful made mustard, if you have no mustard in it already

Use no sugar in the mayonnaise; there are enough forceful flavors without it.

SAUCE TARTARE may be used either for salads, meat, or fish. Cold chicken and tongue, à la Sauce Tartare, is simply delicious.

Make an ordinary mayonnaise, without mustard or sugar. Add to it

> 1 teaspoonful dry mustard
> 2 tablespoonfuls grated onions
> 1 tablespoonful chopped parsley
> A large pinch of cayenne pepper

This chapter could not be considered at all complete if I were to leave it without giving you a word about *egg-thickened sauces*, which are so very much used for rather "good" dishes. A sauce thickened with egg is softer and smoother and more rich than one made with either flour or roux.

It is very generally used for the gravies of delicate meats, — stewed chicken, boiled veal, etc.

Measure into a pan the amount of liquor or gravy that you need, heat it to the boil, and skim it carefully. Take the pan off the fire and let it cool for two minutes. This is very important. A boiling sauce would turn the eggs.

Colette's Best Recipes

The yolk of one egg will thicken half a pint of sauce, but, of course, it would be richer and better if you used two. Pour a little of the hot liquor on the yolks and stir them with a wooden spoon till they are well mixed. Add this mixture to the liquor which remains in the pan, stirring all the while. Set the pan back on a gentle heat, and continue to stir till the sauce thickens. But you must not let it boil, or it will turn.

Never use the white of the egg. It would make lumps and spoil the sauce.

Sauce Poulette

½ pint meat boilings
1 tablespoonful white roux
Salt and red pepper
Yolk of 1 egg

Either a little chopped parsley, or a couple of tablespoonfuls of mushroom, cooked in the meat boilings, and roughly chopped.

Mix as directed above, and add the parsley or mushrooms at the last moment.

SAUCE JAUNE. Make it just like a cream sauce, using the water in which meat or fish has been boiled, in place of milk. When it has cooked for five minutes after thickening, take the pan off the fire and beat in the yolk of an egg. Put the pan back again and stir briskly with a wooden spoon while you count fifty. The fire must be a good, clear one. Now let the sauce cool for five minutes; then stir in two or three tablespoonfuls of vinegar. This is excellent with boiled meat or fish of any kind.

If you want to make good sauces always

Add whatever you may have to add very gradually, stirring all the while. No sauce will stand the addition of a stream of liquid; it must go in drop by drop.

Colette Makes Sauces

Always stir in the same direction; *which* direction does not matter, as long as it is the same one.

If your sauce goes lumpy, put it on a slightly stronger heat than you have used so far and stir it very quickly, trying to beat out the lumps. If they do not disappear almost at once, rub it through a sieve.

If a sauce curdles, it may sometimes be put right if, at the very first sign of the trouble, you throw in a few drops of cold water and stir hard, taking the pan off the fire. But this remedy by no means always succeeds. You could not call it anything better than a last hope for a desperate case.

Keep tasting sauce. Add the seasoning in very small amounts, with a tasting between each. But, though you are so careful not to put in too much of anything, you must remember, all the same, that the meat or vegetable, or whatever it may be, with which the sauce is eaten, will take off from the force of the flavor, so that a sauce which is ideally good when tasted from a spoon, will be poor and *fade* when eaten on meat. So exaggeration in the saucepan means the happy medium on the dish.

Remember, won't you — one is so apt to forget! — that sauces made with meat boilings and fish boilings seldom need the addition of any salt, as it is already in the liquor. If you forget this, and your sauce is too salty, you can nearly always get it right by adding a wee pinch of rough brown sugar; the coarse kind, which is almost like treacle, is best.

CHAPTER XII

COLETTE MAKES CANDIED FRUITS AND SWEETS

IN France, Christmas is nothing like the great social festival that it is in England. As a rule, we keep it rather quietly, reserving all our present-giving and merrymaking for a later date, New Year, when we burst out into sociability of every possible and imaginable kind, and keep it up for a whole week.

During that first week of January, you are bound to call upon all your relations who are within anything like reasonable distance; write to those who are too far off; and give or send presents to every one of them. You also have to call on and give things to all the local lights, such as the curé and the mayor and the doctor; and, worst of all, you have to respond graciously to all the calls and presents and good wishes that are showered upon your defenseless self. A tiring business! But it has its repaying moments, as when the gardener's small, fat grandson, darting out of the stable cottages to catch me as I passed, stammered with breathless earnestness, "Madame! I have the honor to wish you a good year, followed by many others! And good fortune — and good health — and good friends — and — and a good death, followed by many others!"

No doubt about it, it's a tiring business. And it was a very costly one, too, till I discovered that the cheapest way to provide presents for all my "sisters and my

Colette Makes Candied Fruits and Sweets

cousins and my aunts" and their patriotically large families, was to turn Colette loose on sweet-making, and then pack up the results in pretty boxes. She always made sweets very well, and, as each year raises her reputation in the family higher and higher, she becomes more ambitious and does better and better.

It is an understood thing that, at least once in the year, I shall bring her a box of the best candied fruits and bonbons that Paris can produce, and that she shall be allowed to experiment till she can make the same things herself.

The experiments don't always succeed, of course. There are some bonbons which need special molds and colorings, known only to confectioners, and others which can only be made by machine. But she has had a very great number of successes. And I should like, if you will allow me, to pick out for you a dozen or more of those which I consider best of all.

There are just a few technical terms, which are used in *all* French recipes for sweet-making, jam-making, etc., and, if you will have patience with me while I explain them, it will save us a lot of trouble in the future. Would you mind putting a mark in this page, please? I shall use the same terms in other chapters, and I shall not explain them again. They all refer to the preparation of the sugar syrups, in which the fruits are cooked.

MAKING SUGAR SYRUP. Use the best white cane sugar, taking lumps rather than powder. To each pound of sugar allow half a gill of water. Put all into a clean aluminum or copper pan and boil till it reaches the degree indicated in the recipe. Here are the different degrees:

SUGAR "À LISSÉ" (PETIT LISSÉ ET GRAND LISSÉ). Keep a skimmer always in the boiling sugar. Lift up the skimmer, dab your first finger on the sticky edge — where the syrup is so cool that you can touch it quickly without hurting yourself. Press your finger hard on your thumb and separate them immediately and gently.

If an almost imperceptible thread forms between them, breaking instantly, the syrup is cooked to *petit lissé*. If the thread is stronger and longer lasting, the syrup is cooked to *grand lissé*.

SUGAR À PERLÉ — (PETIT PERLÉ, GRAND PERLÉ). Let your sugar cook a little longer and try it in the same way when you see that it is boiling up into round bubbles like beads. If the thread between the finger and thumb stands firm instead of breaking immediately, the syrup is *à perlé*, — *à petit perlé* when it will only bear a slight separation; *à grand perlé* when the hand can be opened quite wide.

SUGAR À SOUFFLÉ AND À LA PLUME. Withdraw your skimmer, which has been boiling in the pan all the time, let it drip a little, and then hold it up and blow through the holes. If you blow little bubbles, which break at once, the syrup is *à soufflé*. If the bubbles stand, lengthening out under your blowing into long or feathery shapes, just as soap bubbles do, the syrup is *à plume*.

SIROP À CASSÉ. Dip your finger and thumb into cold water, then into the boiling sugar; then into cold water again, pressing them hard together. If they stick firm enough to make a breaking sound when they are separated, the syrup is cooked *à cassé*.

SUGAR AU CARAMEL. Bite the little piece of sugar off your fingers. If it sticks to your teeth, it is not yet done; but if it cracks and snaps, it is cooked *au caramel*, and has reached the farthest stage possible in syrup cooking. Take the pan off the fire at once, or it will burn and spoil.

There! That's a long explanation, but it's well worth while, as you will see when we pass on to the recipes. At

Colette Makes Candied Fruits and Sweets

New Year, oranges are about the best and most easily found of fruits, so let us start with them.

ORANGES GLACÉES (SUGARED ORANGES). There are many different kinds of Oranges Glacées. This is the simplest, cheapest, and most quickly done.

Use ripe oranges, taking the kind that have few, if any, pips. Peel them very carefully, removing every scrap of the white skin, and divide them neatly into sections. Now cut little pieces of very fine wire, four or five inches long. Slip a wire along the *small* curve of each section, and twist the ends of the wire so that a ring is formed, by which the fruit can easily be held. Cook a pan of syrup to "*cassé*" and set it on a *very* moderate heat, so that it may stay liquid without cooking too much and turning into toffee. Dip in the pieces of orange one at a time; take them out gently, so that you do not shake off more of the syrup than you can help. Thread the wire rings along a stick or bar, and let the fruit hang till it is dry. Then pull out the wires and arrange the sections in paper frills.

Sections of lemons and limes may be done in the same way. Some people are extremely fond of them, though others find them too sharp. It is a good plan, I think, to coat lemons and limes twice with sugar. You must make a fresh syrup the second time, as the first will go into toffee if you try to reheat it.

By the way, if there is ever some syrup left over from sweet-making, you need not think that it is wasted. Just stew some fruit in the pan; the stewed fruit will be well sweetened, and the pan cleaned at the same time!

ORANGES AU CARAMEL (CARAMELED ORANGES). These are a little more tiresome to do, because the sugar, being cooked to the farthest possible point, is rather inclined to turn to toffee while one is still at work. The best way

Colette's Best Recipes

to avoid this is to boil the syrup in a small pan and stand it inside a big basin of boiling water, so that it may stay liquid without getting any more cooked.

Color the sugar with a drop of carmine. Cook it to "caramel." Have ready your bits of orange, prepared as in the former recipe, and dip and dry them just as before. If you want to make a variation in their appearance, dip them into a bowl of rather coarse crystallized sugar when they have been a few seconds withdrawn from the syrup. The little white spangles on the pink background, with the yellow fruit glinting through, make a charming effect.

Bananas (not too ripe) peeled, cut into rounds about half an inch thick, and carameled in this way are delicious. Don't bother to make wires for them — just spear each up on the end of a fine skewer, dip it, and then tickle it off with another skewer on to a piece of oiled paper, where it must be turned so that it may dry nicely at both sides.

"They know how to make Marrons Glacés in America, don't they?" asked Colette.

"They *make* them," admitted I, "but so folks do in London, you know. And, if the New York marrons are as nasty as the London ones, we shall be doing a good turn by teaching them a different way of setting to work."

MARRONS GLACÉS AU CARAMEL. Prick and roast one pound of chestnuts, taking great care that they do not color. Peel them neatly, trying to remove the inner skins as well as the outer. It is difficult to do this without breaking the nuts, but it can be managed with care. Let them cool. Slip a fine wire into each and make up a ring, just as you did for the pieces of orange. Cook a syrup to *cassé* in a flattish pan. Run the wire rings on little sticks, and lay the sticks from side to side of the pan, so that the nuts may hang in the syrup. Let them remain an hour if, by

Colette Makes Candied Fruits and Sweets

the use of a lower dish of boiling water, you can so long manage to keep the syrup from setting. Then hang them up to dry, just like the oranges.

Those are the real French Marrons Glacés. The things that they call Marrons Glacés in England are really Marrons Confits and are so very troublesome to do and take so long that I should advise any one who can't live without them to overdraw her bank account in buying some ready-made!

VIOLETTES PRALINÉES are not much good to eat — too small — but a stock of them is exceedingly useful to any one who goes in for sweet-making or cake-making. And the Parma violets (so plentiful in Europe and I suppose in America, during winter) are much better for them than the little outdoor kind.

Cut off the stalks. Weigh the flower heads. Cook an equal weight of sugar to *soufflé*, throw in the flower heads, cover the pan, and let it boil one minute. Then pour all into a tin vessel, and let it stand overnight. (The tin helps to keep the natural color in the flowers.)

Next day, reheat all *nearly* to boiling point. Drain out the flowers, lay them on a hair sieve till they won't drip any more.

Color some icing sugar with a little violet coloring worked well into it. Dry it in the oven, sieve it, and roll the flower heads well in it. Lay them on sheets of paper and put them in the rack over the dying fire all night.

ROSES PRALINÉES are done in just the same way, except that fine untinted castor sugar is generally used instead of icing sugar, and that the petals must stand overnight in a china basin instead of a tin one.

I think that the real bonbons are nicer than sugared fruits, as well as being much easier to make.

TRUFFETTES AU CHOCOLAT (CHOCOLATE TRUFFLES) are

Colette's Best Recipes

those very soft chocolates, which melt in your mouth all too soon.

½ pound best fresh butter
¾ pound icing sugar
½ pound of the best unsweetened chocolate, grated fine
2 ounces best sweetened chocolate, grated roughly

Take the first three ingredients, mix them well, and work them with a wooden spoon till the paste is perfectly smooth. Make balls about the size of walnuts, roll them in the roughly grated chocolate, and put them to dry on plates.

That is just the foundation recipe, which may be varied in many different ways.

1. Add a few drops of coffee essence to the chocolate. Many people find this a very great improvement.

2. Put a glacé cherry, or a blanched and grilled almond into the center of each ball.

3. Chop blanched almonds roughly, mix them with the coarse grated chocolate, and roll the balls in them.

4. Coat the balls with desiccated cocoanut, instead of with chocolate.

In any case, remember that, not being cooked at all, they will only keep so long as the butter keeps, — about a week in winter. But they are best when eaten the day they are made. I know one most famous little shop which sells nothing but Truffettes au Chocolat, and will never offer yesterday's wares. They make each morning only as many as they are sure of selling, and, when all are gone, they shut down, — often as early as three in the afternoon.

BONBONS AU CHOCOLAT (CHOCOLATE BONBONS) are very much the same in taste and have the added advantage of keeping well.

Grate quarter of a pound of chocolate finely and put it into a small pan with two tablespoonfuls of milk. Let it

Colette Makes Candied Fruits and Sweets

cook gently for quarter of an hour. Cut six ounces of fresh butter into small pieces and add to the chocolate. While the butter is melting, beat up in a basin the yolks of two eggs, with half a pound of icing sugar. Stir the hot chocolate very well into the eggs and let the whole thing get cold. When it is firm enough to handle, roll it into little bolster shapes, and coat them with roughly grated chocolate.

BONBONS AUX AMANDES (ALMOND BONBONS) are those rough, lumpy goodies which you find in every box of mixed chocolates.

- ¼ pound grated chocolate
- ¼ pound almonds, blanched and roughly chopped
- 3 heaped tablespoonfuls of icing sugar
- 2 tablespoonfuls of coffee essence
- ¾ tablespoonful of fresh butter

Work all together with a wooden spoon, adding either a little more butter or a little more sugar, as required, till you get a paste which is very firm indeed, but not so dry that it breaks. Break it into rough little lumps and roll each in a few more chopped almonds. Let them stand on plates till they are dry.

These sweets gain greatly in appearance by being packed in little frilled papers.

CARAMELS AU CHOCOLAT (CHOCOLATE CARAMELS) are ever so much nicer when made at home than when bought. Those that come from the shops always seem to me to be too hard: but those that Colette makes are dreams of sticky sweetness.

- ½ pound grated chocolate
- 1 gill thick cream
- 1½ ounces of butter
- 3 tablespoonfuls of honey
- 4 heaped tablespoonfuls of sifted sugar

Colette's Best Recipes

Melt the butter, honey, and sugar together in a small pan. Add the cream and stir all on a sharp heat while you count one hundred. Then add the chocolate and keep on stirring till the mixture begins to boil away from the sides of the pan. Try a little bit in cold water. It ought to set so firm that there is a definite something which you can press between your fingers, though it is not nearly so hard as toffee. Pour it out on oiled marble; a marble pastry slab is the best thing. If you have nothing like that, a dish lightly rubbed with olive oil will do. Try to arrange the caramel so that it hardens into a sheet about half an inch thick. When it is nearly cold, cut it with a sharp knife which has been rubbed over with a little oil. Let the caramels go quite cold before you wrap each in a wee twist of waxed paper.

It is rather hard to cut them without getting the edges ragged, but if you use a heavy knife, not too sharp, oiling it lightly and *sawing* with it, rather than making strokes, you will manage nicely, I feel sure.

CARAMELS AU CAFÉ (COFFEE CARAMELS) have a very delicious flavor, but I do not like the texture of them quite as much as that of the chocolate ones. Unless you are very careful in the boiling, they are inclined to turn into coffee toffee, which, though an excellent thing in its own way, is *not* caramel.

        1 pound castor sugar
        6 ounces of fresh butter
        1 gill fresh cream
        1 gill very strong black coffee

Boil the sugar and butter together for ten minutes, stirring carefully. Add the coffee and cream and go on stirring for ten minutes more. Then start trying the prepa-

Colette Makes Candied Fruits and Sweets

ration in cold water. Finish it off just like the chocolate caramels.

Dattes Fourées (Stuffed Dates)

¼ pound ground almonds
¼ pound icing sugar
2 ounces of pistachio nuts, chopped fairly fine
A little "sirop à cassé" (see page 140)

Pound the almonds and sugar together till they are very well mixed. Add the pistachio nuts and enough syrup to bind the whole to a paste. Split the dates down one side, stone them, stuff them with little balls of the paste, and close them carefully. Have ready a pan of syrup cooked *à cassé*. Stick a knitting needle into each date, dip it in the syrup, and then use another knitting needle to tickle it off on to a lightly oiled dish. Leave them till dry. The coating of sugar will be very thick and quite transparent, so that it will not at all rob the dates of their characteristic appearance.

French plums may be stuffed in the same way, — I mean those bluish plums, which are sold in flat wooden boxes. Stuffing them is a profitable sort of job for the stuffer, because their stones have already been replaced by a plug of fruit, and you have to take this out before you can put the nut mixture in. And, once out, obviously it has no other use in the world but to be eaten at once!

KLONGAS is very much indeed like Chocolate Caramels but rather harder. It is very often given to children, as it is both nourishing and wholesome.

1 quart good cream
1 pound castor sugar
½ pound grated chocolate

Cook on a gentle heat till the chocolate and sugar have melted. Then move the pan to a very hot place and stir hard all the while with a wooden spoon, till a drop of the mixture sets at once when it is put into cold water. It should fall heavily to the bottom of the water and set firm, like toffee. Finish it off just like caramels.

MASSEPAINS are dull alone, I think. But Colette often makes them very wee, and, when they are cold, coats them with Truffette au Chocolat mixture. Then they become perfectly delicious. You can very well make them up in those big blocks — about one and a half inches each way — which are wrapped in silver paper, and called Bouchées, though I should be very sorry, myself, to be obliged to take a whole one at a mouthful!

½ pound ground sweet almonds
1 ounce ground bitter almonds
½ pound icing sugar
The whites of two eggs
A few drops of flavoring if you like, though most people find that the almonds alone have flavor enough

Beat the whites of the eggs to a stiff froth. Add the almonds first, working them well in with your fingers, and then the sugar, — or as much of it as the paste will take without getting too dry. Knead it very well indeed, just like bread. Make it into any shapes you like, put them on oiled paper, and bake them quarter of an hour in a very gentle oven.

Let them cool. Then either eat them plain, or coat them as I told you above.

NOUGAT DE MONTÉLIMAR is very good indeed, as every one knows, and worth the trouble that it takes to make. But don't try it unless you can buy rice paper with which to cover it while it cools, for it goes so horribly sticky and messy if you try to make it without any.

You will want a large, square shaped tin of some kind,

Colette Makes Candied Fruits and Sweets

which can be lined at bottom and sides with two thicknesses of rice paper. Prepare this beforehand.

Now take two pounds of the best honey and boil it *au petit cassé*, stirring it most carefully all the while with a wooden spoon. Beat the whites of four eggs to the stiffest possible froth and stir them in. Put the pan on a more gentle heat and keep stirring constantly. If you are not very careful indeed, it may suddenly puff up and all go over the sides. Go on cooking till the mixture is again at *cassé*. Now stir in two pounds of almonds, which have been blanched, dried, and cut into slips. Pour out the nougat into your prepared tin, letting it lie, if possible, about one and a half to two inches deep. Smooth out another sheet of rice paper flat on top. Leave it till it is quite cool.

Now comes the awful moment! Your block will come out of the tin quite easily, and look innocent and good enough. But, when you try to cut it into bars or squares, you'll find that you have caught a Tartar. It sticks to everything! Especially to you! And the better it is, the more it sticks; it's a sign of good nougat to be sticky. So you can't even comfort yourself by blaming it. But by the help of courage, a very sharp knife dipped in boiling water and then dried quickly, and lots of rice paper in which to fold the detached pieces, you may arrive at a happy result, — perhaps.

If you want to make good bonbons always

1. Get all your odds and ends ready beforehand — almonds blanched, chocolate grated, and so on — so that you may have them all at hand, and not be distracted from your bonbons at the critical moment of cooking.

2. **Keep your** bonbon pan strictly for that alone. All these sugary things are just waiting for an excuse to burn,

and you will certainly give it to them if you use a pan in which other things have been cooked.

3. Dry blanched almonds, and even brown them in the oven. If you use them fresh and soft, they turn musty almost at once.

4. Buy the very best sugar and the very best chocolate that can be got for money. Let the chocolate be perfectly plain, unsweetened cooking chocolate, but of a very high quality. Never get it from a confectioner, but, if you cannot deal with the factory direct, at least go to a very big and reliable grocery store. If you use cocoa instead of chocolate, increase the amount of sugar in the recipe by one fifth, and add a pinch of powdered cinnamon, to soften the harsh flavor of the cocoa.

CHAPTER XIII

COLETTE MAKES CAKES AND BISCUITS

"GOOD Americans, when they die, go to Paris," runs the saying.

I don't know about that. But, whatever they may do when they are dead, they certainly go to Paris in astonishing numbers while they are alive. And it is for them, and also for the English visitors, that a multitude of smart tea shops have been opened in all the best streets. They are called "Five-o'clocks", though, of course, nobody ever dreams of going there at five. When you lunch between eleven and twelve, you begin to want your tea somewhere around 3.30 P.M.

Last time I went on a shopping trip to Paris, I took Colette with me, because she needed new spectacles. Thinking to give her a treat, I took her to tea at a Five-o'clock, one day. But it was not a success. Colette "passed remarks" in a loud voice on every bun she ate, and, finally, almost wept when she discovered that I was going to pay ten francs for our entertainment.

"Ten francs!" wailed she, blocking up the road to the pay desk with her stout and agitated old figure. "But it is a crime that — a real crime! Ten francs for a cup of coffee that one drinks in a single swallow, so small is it, and half a dozen little nothings that have the impertinence to call themselves cakes. Cakes, indeed! As if it was only

Colette's Best Recipes

in Paris that such cakes could make themselves! Give me a couple of eggs and a little sugar — !"

"I'll give you anything you like if you'll only hush and come away," whispered I, desperately tugging at her arm. So out we bundled, followed by a wave of admiring giggles and whispers. I would have shaken Colette if I could have found a private corner to do it in, and if she had not been so heavy! But, all the same, there was truth in what she said; these little fancy cakes, which one gets in confectioners' shops, are a plain steal. If you make them at home you will get about twenty for the price that one would cost you in the shop. And they really are not difficult to do, when once you know how.

Let me tell you the "how" of just a few.

In the first place, I wonder if your oven has a top heat? A coal-range oven, which is worth anything at all, heats itself naturally at the top as well as at the bottom; but gas and electric ovens, which have only bottom heats, are not very good for cake baking. Your little things get burned underneath, while they stay pale and dull on the upper side. What you want is a row of gas or electric jets along the oven roof, from which the heat will beat *down* on to your cakes, as well as one from which it will beat *up*; and, in France at least, you can generally get an oven like that to your gas stove if you make fuss enough about it.

But, if your stove is fixed already, and you can do nothing, you must make the best of a bad job by heating it very carefully before you start, and then fixing the pressure so that the temperature stays steady. It is sheer foolishness, and waste of time and materials, to stoke up the fire or turn up the gas after the cake is in, thinking that, so long as the heat gets to work one time or another, it does not much matter when. A good heat is nearly always wanted

Colette Makes Cakes and Biscuits

at the start to make the cake rise. (There are a few exceptions, but that's the general rule.) And, if it does not get its chance to rise in the first few minutes, the outside will be toughened into a swell-proof crust, and the unfortunate cake will be ruined beyond praying for.

Always test your oven before using it. (I once bought Colette an oven thermometer in a wooden frame, which, rather to my surprise, she received with warm thanks. She hung it outside the kitchen window and tapped it industriously, and, after a few days of useless effort, was rather stiff with me on the subject of the very inferior weatherglass I had given her!) This is how she tests her oven. And a very good way, too.

When the oven is all heated, put into the hottest place a sheet of ordinary thin writing paper. Shut the door. Count one hundred. Then look at the result.

If the paper is *blackened and smelling*, the oven is *fierce* — right for pastry, bread, and a few cakes.

If the paper is *deeply browned*, the oven is *brisk*, — right for the majority of small buns and some biscuits.

If the paper is *pale brown*, the oven is *moderate*, — right for sponge cakes and the majority of biscuits.

If the paper is a little crisped but *not colored at all*, the oven is *slow*, — right for meringues, and other things that just have to be dried gradually.

There's a lot more to say, but I think I'll put it in the list at the end of the chapter. Just turn that up and study it, won't you, before you try any of the recipes?

BISCUITS À LA CUILLER. Break the yolks of five eggs into one basin and the whites into another. Add to the yolks three quarters of a pound of sifted sugar, and beat them with a wooden spoon steadily for half an hour, till you get a cream that is white and thick. Stir in very

Colette's Best Recipes

gently one quarter of a pound of flour and a teaspoon of orange-flower water. Whip up the whites to a froth so stiff that it will support a whole egg, and fold it into the mixture as gently as ever you can. Have ready a baking tin covered with buttered paper. Take a teaspoon of the mixture. Lay the point of the spoon on the paper and then gently draw it backward, letting the mixture trickle out as you go, till you have a bar about three inches long. Cover the paper with these bars. Sift a little sugar over them and bake them in a very moderate oven till they are set and a very delicate brown.

Are they like sponge biscuits? Yes. They're the same with a big difference.

In all the dessert recipes for which I have recommended you to use sponge cakes, Biscuits à la Cuiller will do as well, or better. Colette makes up a lot at a time, and stores them in a tin, so that she may always have them at hand for desserts.

ALMOND MERINGUES. Beat up the white of an egg, and while you are beating it, sift into it three ounces of powdered sugar. Keep on beating till you have a froth. Then put the basin containing it into a pan of boiling water, and let the water boil around the basin while you keep on beating for fifteen minutes. Take the basin out of the pan, add twenty almonds, blanched and chopped, and a teaspoon of coffee essence. Sprinkle a baking tin lightly with flour, and pile the mixture on it in little high lumps, leaving good spaces between them, as they will spread in baking. Cook in a gentle oven till set, and cool on a cake wire. These meringues are very nice indeed without cream filling which may be added if desired.

CHOCOLATE MERINGUES. Beat the whites of two eggs to a very stiff froth and stir in gently one bar of grated

Colette Makes Cakes and Biscuits

chocolate and six tablespoons of sugar. Cover a baking sheet with paper and sugar it lightly. Drop the mixture on it, a tablespoon at a time, leaving a good space between them, and taking care to get them as nearly alike in shape as possible. Sprinkle them lightly with sugar and put them into a gentle oven till they are set. Lift them up carefully, scoop out the soft underneath part of each, turn them on their backs on a clean sheet of paper, and put them back again in the oven to dry. Fill them with whipped cream when they are cold, and clap them together in pairs. Delicious! Much nicer than plain sugar meringues!

ALMOND CHAINS. Melt three quarters of a pound of butter in a good sized basin. Stir into it three quarters of a pound of sifted sugar. Then beat in three eggs, one at a time, giving a good brisk beating to each, and, finally, work in enough flour to make a paste of the consistency of putty. Blanch and chop finely one half pound of almonds and work them well into the paste. Take a little piece at a time — covering the lump with a damp cloth to keep it from hardening — roll your piece out as fine as possible, cut it into tiny narrow strips with a sharp knife, and roll these strips into little rings, pinching the ends. Fasten one ring through another till you have a chain. Bake on a buttered tin in an oven quickly enough to color the rings lightly. Take the chain out of the oven with the greatest possible care.

You can make nice little biscuits by cutting the same paste into ordinary round or finger shapes. The chains are rather bothersome to make, but they are very pretty, and, for a children's party, or anything of that sort, they are a novelty perfectly certain to score a success, when used for table decoration.

CHOCOLATE CROQUETTES. Take three quarters of a

pound of powdered sugar, three bars of grated chocolate and two whites of eggs. Put them all together into a basin and stir with a small wooden spoon for one half hour, stirring always in the same direction round and round. You need not beat hard; just keep on stirring. Rub a little oil on to a sheet of paper, spread it on the baking sheet, and drop the mixture on it in small drops or bars, remembering that they must have room to spread a good deal. Bake five to seven minutes in a gentle oven. Cool on a cake wire. They will become quite crisp.

CARDINAL'S CAKE. Bring a breakfast cup of milk to the boil, sweeten it well, and flavor it with vanilla. Beat together three eggs and six tablespoons of flour till they are well mixed, stir in the milk just as it is boiling up into foam. Pour all into a well-buttered mold and put into a quick oven for fifteen minutes. Loosen the cake with a knife, turn it out on a hot plate and serve it at once.

What is it like? Well, it's a cross between a soufflé and a very light batter cake. It must be eaten hot, because it toughens when it gets cold. But it won't have any chance to stay and cool — too good!

CHESTNUT CAKE. Take thirty chestnuts, boil them till tender and slip them out of their skins. Mix into them one quarter of a pound of powdered sugar, one quarter of a pound of melted butter, the yolks of four eggs, and a few drops of vanilla. Beat the whites of the eggs to a very stiff froth and stir it in gently. Butter a plain tin of the size for a three-pound cake and sprinkle it with as much flour as will stick to the buttered sides. Cook the cake for three quarters of an hour in a steady but not too quick oven. Try it by thrusting a straw into the thickest part. If the straw comes out clean, the cake is done.

Let it get cold. Sprinkle with sugar or pile it with

Colette Makes Cakes and Biscuits

little mounds of whipped cream. Use a very sharp knife to cut it, as it is so light.

Quatre-quarts

4 eggs
Their weight in flour, sifted sugar, and butter
The juice of 1 lemon
2 ounces blanched almonds

Separate the yolks and whites of the eggs. Put the yolks into a basin with the sugar, the flour, the melted butter, and the lemon juice. Stir with a wooden spoon till the cream becomes white and light (about fifteen minutes). Add a grain of salt to the whites and whip them till a fork stuck in them will stand upright. Fold the whites into the yellow mixture as gently as ever you can.

Have ready a plain cake tin, buttered with fresh butter, and sprinkled over with a little flour and sifted sugar. Fill it not more than half full. Sprinkle the top of the cake with the almonds, blanched and chopped. Start it in a moderate oven and move it to a cooler place if you see that it is getting too much colored. It ought to take about an hour to cook.

Try it by thrusting a straw into the center. If the straw comes out clean, the cake is done.

It is a sort of sponge cake, and Colette thinks more highly of it than of the real French sponge cake, which is called Biscuit de Savoie, which is horribly lengthy and difficult to make, and not particularly good when it is done. Quatre-quarts is just as light and wholesome as Biscuit de Savoie, and it keeps much better, because there is a little butter in it.

CHOUX À LA CRÈME (CREAM PUFFS). In England, folks put coffee or chocolate icing on them and call them éclairs. But it is all the same thing.

Make the paste for which the recipe is given under the

Colette's Best Recipes

name of Pets de Nonne (page 106). Cover the oven sheet with buttered paper and drop on it little lumps of paste, each the size of a walnut. Leave a couple of inches between each. Brush them over with the beaten yolk of an egg and let them stand twenty minutes before putting them into the oven. They want a brisk heat to make them rise. You must not open the oven door, or down they will go with a flop, as the cold air rushes in and presses on them. Stand near and sniff hard. As soon as you can smell baking, open the door, powder them thickly with fine sugar, and put them back again, so that they may go glacé. After two minutes, take them out and cool them on a sieve. Just before serving, slit each at the side and fill it with whipped cream.

Sometimes they are sprinkled with chopped almonds instead of powdered sugar; then a little strawberry jam is whipped up with the cream.

If you want to make éclairs, put the paste through a forcing bag or tube of stiff paper, so that you can arrange it in bars about the size of your middle finger. When they are quite cold, ice them with a simple chocolate or coffee icing.

CHOCOLATE ICING. Melt three ounces icing sugar, and two ounces grated chocolate in three tablespoonfuls of boiling water. Warm the icing till it is perfectly liquid, but *don't let it boil.* Hold each éclair in turn over the pan and trickle the mixture on it with a spoon. Don't touch them till they are quite cold and dry.

Coffee Icing

4 ounces sugar
2 tablespoonfuls coffee essence
2 tablespoonfuls boiling water

Make as above.

Colette Makes Cakes and Biscuits

SAINT HONORÉ is a sort of traditional French cake, just like the traditional English plum cake.

Make the same paste as for Choux à la Crème, and form rather more than three quarters of it into a large round, the thickness of your little finger. Cut it with the edge of a saucepan lid, to make it neat.

Divide the rest of the paste into very wee balls, not larger than marbles, and put them on buttered paper. Bake all in a hot oven. The little balls will only take a few minutes and should be glacéd as thickly as possible; the big cake will take nearly one half hour and should be left plain.

When both are cold, make a wall of little balls all around the edge of the big cake, alternating them with different kinds of glacé fruits here and there, and sticking both fruit and balls into place by dabs of jam or syrup. Just before serving, pile the middle of the cake with whipped cream and decorate it with more fruits. Or, if you prefer, you may flavor the cream with coffee or chocolate and use no fruits at all.

BABAS are those tall, light buns, soaked in rum, which are as common in Paris as penny buns in London. If you don't care to use rum, a sugar syrup, with a few drops of any strong fruit essence in it, will do well.

$\frac{1}{2}$ pound flour
$\frac{1}{2}$ ounce dry yeast

Mix the yeast into three tablespoonfuls water. When it is well mixed, add enough flour to make a firm paste and work this paste with your fingers to a smooth ball. Put the ball into a large basin; cover it with the rest of the flour; spread a clean towel over all and set the basin in a warm, but not hot, place for five hours.

"I put it on a chair at the side of the fire," Colette says.

Colette's Best Recipes

"Not right in front, you know, as if it were clothes to air; but just at the side, where I might sit comfortably myself."

At the end of five hours, take out the yeast ball — which will be much swollen — and mix up the flour which remains with four tablespoonfuls of milk, one teaspoonful salt, and one quarter of a pound of good butter. Work all with your hands into a smooth paste; add an egg and work it well in; when it is no longer visible, add another and do the same with that.

Now add the yeast ball, one quarter pound sugar, a wine glassful of rum or fruit syrup, and one quarter pound seeded raisins, and give all a final working. It is important that the whole should be well and evenly mixed, but don't work it more than is necessary; the less of hand that it gets at this stage, the lighter it will be.

Grease some of those little, tall cake tins, which are used for Castle Puddings. (If you have n't any of that shape, never mind: the Babas will taste just as good if they come out square or round, though, of course, they won't look right.) Fill the tins rather less than half full and set them in a warm place till the dough rises up so much that it fills them. Then bake in a quick oven till nicely browned and try them with a straw, just as you do all buns. Tap them out of their tins on to a cake wire, and, as soon as they are cool, soak them in rum or fruit syrup. Let them drip all they can before you serve them.

I have spent a lot of time and trouble telling you about Babas, but I think it is worth while, because, in very much the same way are made two more famous French cakes, — Brioche and Savarin. They are not very generally made in French town households, where the baker in every street is sure to sell them; but no big country house would dream

Colette Makes Cakes and Biscuits

of accepting a cook who was not well up in all three, and prepared to make them on baking days.

BRIOCHE. Make exactly like the Baba till you come to the adding of the raisins, rum, etc. *Don't add these,* — neither raisins, nor rum, nor anything else. Just leave the paste quite plain, work the yeast ball into it lightly. Throw a clean towel over the empty basin, lay the lump of dough lightly on the towel. If you want a simple Brioche, you can color it with a pinch of saffron, and use four tablespoonfuls of milk to replace the eggs.

"And keep pulling the cloth, till you make the dough hang as if it were in a hammock," says Colette. "The air must be able to get to it underneath, as well as on top."

Throw another cloth over it and leave it in a cool place all night.

When the oven is heated as much as possible for baking, flatten out your Brioche paste on a floured board. Take the four corners, and bring them in to the middle. Turn the lump over, so that the corners are underneath, flatten it out again. Repeat the whole process four times.

Take a little bit of your paste to make the head of the brioche. Put the rest into a buttered, fluted tin, — one of those cake tins which makes a much bigger circle at the top than at the bottom. It should not be more than half full. Stick on the head with a little drop of water and put the Brioche into the hottest possible oven. Cover it with a sheet of buttered paper if it goes too brown.

It will take about one hour to cook, — one half an hour in the sharp heat, and the second half in a more moderate place.

You can tell if it is done by turning it out of the tin, and tapping the bottom crust sharply. If it rings clear, it is done right through; if it rings dull, there is still uncooked matter towards the middle.

Colette's Best Recipes

Brioches may be made tiny and are easier to bake like this than when they are big. Put tiny ones in rough dabs on a sheet of buttered paper and let them rise as they will.

SAVARIN can't be made without a special tin in which to bake it. It must be a large round, with a hole in the middle; no other shape will do. But maybe you have a tin like that; it is not an uncommon shape.

Make the yeast ball, as for the Baba, and let it rise in the flour. Then take it out and put it into a basin with

    1 gill milk
    ¼ pound sifted sugar
    ¼ pound melted butter
    1 egg, beaten just enough to mix the yolk and white
    As much salt as will lie on the nail of your little finger

Beat all together *with your hand* till the mixture feels light and frothy. *A spoon cannot be used.* Add the rest of the flour gradually.

Butter the tin and coat it as thickly as you can with almonds, blanched and chopped. Fill the tin half full only with the paste and stand it in a warm place for four hours. The rack above the stove, in between meals, when the fire is low, is about the best place for it.

The paste ought to rise right up, so that it laps the edges of the tin. When it has done this, sprinkle it with almonds, put it into a very hot oven, and bake it just like the Brioche. Cool it on a cake wire and soak it with rum or fruit syrup, just like the Baba.

"That's enough of those big, important, national cakes," say I. "Now give them some nice, little, simple things, Colette, something that they can just toss together in a few minutes when friends come to tea."

Biscômes

½ pound honey   5 ounces almonds, blanched and chopped
2 ounces sugar   A small half teaspoonful powdered cinnamon

Colette Makes Cakes and Biscuits

Mix all together with your hand and work in enough flour to make a paste so firm that it leaves the fingers clean. Keep on kneading till it is soft and pliable. Roll it out to paper thickness, stamp it with a tumbler or round biscuit cutter. Bake the Biscômes on a buttered tin in a brisk oven till they are well browned. Put them on a cake wire just for a moment, so that they may crisp, but serve them while they are still warm. They are the crackliest, crispiest honey biscuits that any one could wish to eat.

Colmoriennes
½ pound sugar, melted in the juice of an orange
¾ pound flour
5 ounces butter, melted till it is most creamy, but not oily

Stir all these well together and add as much more flour as is necessary to make a paste which is just firm enough to handle, but not at all dry or breakable. Roll out this paste very thin and cut it with a wine glass or biscuit cutter. Bake it like the Biscômes.

These little biscuits keep well and are very useful for handing with stewed fruit, rich creams, or anything of that kind.

COPEAUX (SHAVINGS) do look exactly like wood shavings, when they are nicely made. The right way to serve them is to pile them up in a basket lined with lace paper.

5 ounces sugar
6 ounces flour
2 eggs
A few drops of vanilla flavoring

Beat the eggs till they are just well mixed. Add the sugar and beat for three minutes more. Now put in the vanilla, and then the flour, little by little, beating all the while. You ought to get a soft paste, which is just firm enough to roll out. Roll it to tissue-paper thinness and

Colette's Best Recipes

cut it into strips which are one half inch wide and as long as your oven sheet. Butter the oven sheet, lay the strips on it without letting them touch each other, and cook in a very hot oven.

They will color almost at once. Take them up one by one, leaving the rest in a place where they will keep warm and therefore soft. Have ready a smooth stick — a hoop stick does well — with just a very little butter rubbed on it to make it slippy. Twist each band lightly round the stick and let it remain a moment, so that it may set and harden into curls, like those of a shaving. Slip it off as soon as it is set and leave it on a cake wire to crisp.

FRIANDS AUX POMMES DE TERRE (POTATO DAINTIES). They are very much like doughnuts, I believe. (Not that my acquaintance with doughnuts is extensive!) They are awfully good, and very cheap. Only you must eat them hot; they are no use when they get cold.

Boil a pound of potatoes in their skins. Peel them, put them through a sieve, and mix them with quarter of a teaspoonful salt and enough flour to bind the whole into a smooth paste. Work it with your fists. Put your whole strength into it and go at it hard till you feel as if you were kneading butter. Then pat the paste out into little round cakes about the size of —

"Colette, what size is a dollar?"

"How should I know — never seen one."

"No more have I. Lots of dollar checks, but never the real article. And, maybe, those folks over there have never seen an English five-shilling piece; and a franc is too small."

"Tell them to make their Friands the size of a wrist watch. Every one has a wrist watch," says the resourceful Colette.

Colette Makes Cakes and Biscuits

— the size of a wrist watch, drop them into deep fat which is heated to smoking point, and fry them till they turn brown and swim. Drain them out. Slip the point of a knife into the side of each, pass in a little hot jam by the cut, roll them in sifted sugar, and serve at once.

Jam — any sort you like — but nothing made with lemons or oranges! For some reason which I don't know, these two flavors are absolutely loathsome when you get them mixed in with fried potato.

GATEAU FÉCULE (CORNSTARCH CAKE) is a sort of soufflé, with just enough cornstarch in it to stick it together. It is a fine thing for an invalid, who has been ordered to eat lots of eggs.

Take six eggs and separate the whites from the yolks. Add a grain of salt to the whites and whip them to a foam so stiff that a fork can stand in it. Whip the yolks till they are so well beaten that they change from a yellow liquid to a pale cream. Mix together a tablespoonful of cornstarch (heaped up) and a tablespoonful of powdered sugar. Mix the whites and yolks together and keep on whipping lightly while you let the starch and sugar fall in like rain.

Have ready a buttered mold "and cook the cake in a gay oven," says Colette. "That is to say, one that is just midway between moderate and brisk. Turn it out on a cake wire to cool — and mind you don't break it."

If you want to make good cakes *always*

1. Sift and dry the flour before you use it. Damp flour makes heavy cakes.

2. Wring the butter in a clean cloth, to take out the water. Watery butter makes cakes that are heavy and biscuits that are tough.

3. Do all your mixing in a *warm* place, unless the recipe says something different.

Colette's Best Recipes

4. Try to get into the way of beating and stirring always in the same direction, round and round the bowl. I don't say that a cake which is beaten around and across and up and down is going to be a bad cake for that reason: but it will be less perfect in texture, and probably a little less light than one which is always beaten in the same direction.

5. When whites of eggs have been whipped separately and then folded in, remember that you must not beat the mixture more than you can help after they have been added. Beating *before* gets air into the cake, and makes it puff nicely. Beating *after* smashes the air out of the whites and makes them no good at all.

6. Always heat and test your oven the way I have told you.

7. Never open the oven door while the cakes are in, if you can help it, as the inrush of cold air keeps them from rising.

8. Never grease cake tins with either margarine or salt butter, for both make the cakes stick and burn. Fresh butter, or a little good lard are the best things.

9. If you have no good grease, line the tin with four thicknesses of plain white paper, — nothing else at all. You'll find that the cake bakes beautifully and that, though the inside thickness of paper sticks, it can very easily be damped off when the cake is cold.

10. If cakes or buns burn to the tin, put a cloth wet with cold water under them, and let them stay for five minutes. You will find that they then come loose without breaking.

11. If cakes and buns are burned, don't scrape them with a knife. Let them get quite cold and then grate off the black gently with a nutmeg grater. Sprinkle a little

Colette Makes Cakes and Biscuits

sifted sugar over the place, and no one will notice that there has been anything wrong.

12. If you want cakes or buns to keep fresh a long while, put half of an apple in the tin with them. But never do this with biscuits, as it would turn them limp at once.

13. If your oven is too fierce at the bottom, stand a shallow pan of silver sand on the shelf, and plant the cake tins in this. Another very good plan is to keep two or three bricks in the oven and stand the tins on them, thus allowing the hot air to circulate right round the cakes.

You will notice that there is no baking powder in any of these recipes. It is a modern invention, at which Colette turns up her old nose! And it is quite true that you don't need baking powder if you are prepared to spend hours in whipping your eggs almost stiff before you use them. But, if you happen to be in a hurry, and you want to make things go well with less beating, you will generally find it a good plan to mix into the flour as much baking powder as will lie on the nail of your first finger, — *not more*. So many cooks make the mistake of slamming in baking powder by the tablespoonful. And then they complain of the nasty, flat, soda taste which spoils their baking. What else can they expect? The yeast cakes, meringues, and the Gateau Fécule must not have baking powder put into them on any account.

CHAPTER XIV

COLETTE COOKS FRUIT

BEHIND this old, gray-stone house, the fruit gardens and orchard go sloping gently down to the river. Long ago, when we were all at home, and the place was really kept up, the fruit gardens were, I remember "a sight to see", of which my father was justly proud; and Colette is never tired of "talking tall" about the fruit she used to have for her compotes and jams.

The gardens are a wilderness now, for if old Albert manages to keep the front rose beds tidy, that's all I can ask of him. But they still yield fruit in such abundance that we don't know how to pick it. And, if the apples and strawberries are a little less fine than they were in the bygone days for which Colette mourns, what does that matter? They are all the same size when they are eaten, I tell her.

And eaten they do get, in astonishingly large quantities, too. For Colette loves cooking fruit and does it in so many dainty ways that it is difficult to pick out the best. I have tried to choose those that are peculiar to French cookery; and I shall be quite disappointed if the majority of them are not novelties to you.

POMMES FLAMBANTES (APPLE BONFIRE). Allow two moderate-sized apples for each person. Peel and core them without breaking them. Put them into a flat pan, in which they can all stand on the bottom, and add a tea-

Colette Cooks Fruit

cupful of water, three quarters of a teacupful of sugar and a stick of cinnamon. Stew gently till the apples are tender, turning them, if necessary, so that they may cook on both sides. Take them out and drain them carefully. Pile them up on a fireproof dish and keep them very warm. Boil the syrup fast, with the lid off the pan, till it is thick and sticky. Pour it over the apples and powder them thickly with sugar. Just before serving the dish, set light to it with a drop of spirit. You only need a spoonful or two, just to start the fire, and make the whole pile flare up in a most effective way. Serve it while it still flares, just like an English Plum Pudding.

MARMELADE DE POMMES (APPLE MARMALADE). Take eight apples of moderate size, peel them, quarter them, take away the cores, and put them into a pan with quarter pound sugar, one tablespoonful butter, two tablespoonfuls water. Cook very gently, stirring often, so that the fruit may not stick and scorch, which it readily does. When it has stewed quite soft, put it through a sieve, smooth it neatly into a dish, sprinkle it with sugar, and brown it, either with an iron or under the grill. Garnish it liberally with tiny triangles of bread fried in butter.

POMMES AU BEURRE (BUTTERED APPLES) is a sort of standard dish with us, just as, I gather, apple pie is with you.

Take good cooking apples, peel them and core them without breaking them. Cut small thick pieces of the white of bread and stand one apple on each in a fireproof dish. Take a small piece of butter, roll it in as much sugar as it will pick up, and stuff each apple with this. Set the dish in a moderate oven for ten minutes. Then stuff the apples with more butter and sugar, and, till they are done, baste them frequently with the liquid that trickles into the dish. When cooked, they should be tender, but not baked to a

Colette's Best Recipes

mash. Serve either hot or cold in *the dish in which they were baked*. The brown "cracky bits" around the edge are far too nice to be wasted by a change of dishes.

POMMES PORTUGAISES (PORTUGUESE APPLES) are made by filling Pommes au Beurre with hot apricot jam, just at the moment of service.

CROÛTES AUX POMMES (APPLES WITH FRIED BREAD) is a very fine way of using up windfall fruit, which is always rather sour and tasteless unless it gets something to help it out.

Peel the fruit, cut it up any way you like, and cook it in plain water till it is quite tender. Drain it. Mash it through a sieve. Now add one small pot of red currant jelly for each two cups of apple, and sugar to taste. Reheat all and pour it over small squares of bread, fried in butter.

All kinds of stewed fruit may be served in this way; that is to say, all kinds may be poured over slices of fried bread and served hot. But apple is the only one that needs to have jelly added to it; the others are best cooked plain, in a sugar and water syrup.

POMMES MERINGUES (APPLE MERINGUE). Peel, core, and slice your apples. Weigh one pound of them after they have been sliced. Put them into a pan with quarter of a pound of butter and half a pound of sugar and cook them gently till tender. (The thinner the slices in which they are cut, the quicker and more satisfactory the cooking will be). Pile them up on a dish in the tallest pyramid that you can manage. Beat the whites of four eggs to a froth so stiff that a fork will stand in it. Fold in gently two tablespoonfuls of powdered sugar. Coat the fruit with the meringue and set the dish in a good oven till it is just tinted. Serve at once.

Colette Cooks Fruit

Pears may be served in the same way, but they are generally thought less nice than apples.

POMMES RÉGENCE (ROYALTY APPLES). Stew one pound of apples in plain water. When they are soft, drain them, put them through a sieve, and add sugar to taste, with enough of their own water to reduce the mixture to the consistency of a thick purée. Beat in the yolks of three eggs and put the mixture into a buttered pie dish,—a round one is prettiest. The dish should not be more than half full. Spread a generous layer of red currant jelly on the apples. Whip the whites of the three eggs to a very stiff froth, adding a little sifted sugar. Pile this on the jelly. Color the whole thing in a good oven and serve either hot or cold.

You should keep a piece of paper laid over this pudding at first, or the whites will get burned before the inside is cooked enough. It should remain in the oven for twenty minutes all together.

This is one of the best ways of using dried apples, which, if carefully stewed, seem almost exactly like fresh ones.

POMMES À LA CRÈME (CREAMED APPLES) looks pretty, and is very nice for children.

Take custard cups, or small, pretty saucers, and fit each with an apple which is just large enough to go in nicely, leaving space for a little liquid around it. Peel and core the apples without breaking them and stew them gently, taking care that they do not go to pulp. Plenty of sugar should be used in the stewing, but not too much water. When they are cooked, drain them out and put each into its cup. Measure the syrup that remains and make about the same amount of *very* thick custard-powder custard. When both syrup and custard are cool, but not yet quite cold, beat them well together and pour them around the apples. Decorate the cups with scraps of pink and green glacé fruits and set them on ice till the moment of service.

POMMES OU POIRES AU RIZ (APPLES OR PEARS WITH RICE). Wash quarter pound of rice carefully and put it on to boil with two ounces of sugar and just enough water to cover it. Let it cook steadily for three quarters of an hour, adding a little more water if necessary, and shaking the pan to keep the rice from sticking. It should cook itself into a thick, soft mass.

Turn this mash out on a glass dish and let it get cold. When it is quite cold, decorate it with the halves of pears or apples, neatly peeled and stewed. Boil the fruit syrup till it becomes thick and sticky, add a drop of pink coloring to make it pretty, and pour it over all.

A little whipped cream, piled on the fruit, is a great improvement.

COMPOTE DE POIRES (STEWED PEARS) in France are always left whole, unless they are windfalls, which have got badly knocked about, and then excuses are made for serving them in a cut-up state. The correct thing is to peel them neatly, leaving the stalks, put them into a pan with sugar and water just enough to cover them, and a tablespoonful of vinegar, which turns them pink. Stew them slowly and steadily till they are quite tender. Then take them out and arrange them in a glass dish, with all their stalks meeting at the middle and the pears themselves standing on their heads. Boil the syrup fast, with the lid off the pan, till it grows thick and sticky; then strain it over the fruit and serve all cold.

POIRES AU FOUR (BAKED PEARS) are very popular also. The large winter kinds are generally used for baking. Wipe them well and put them into a fairly good oven. Watch them carefully and, if you see any signs of burning, move them to a cooler place; but a very slack heat will not do for them, any more than it will for baked potatoes. They take from one and a half to three hours to cook, according to their kind and size. Test them with a knitting needle. Serve them very hot and hand sugar with them, as of course they have not been sugared at all.

COMPOTE RÔTI (COMPOTE OF ROAST PEARS) is very nice, and quite a change from ordinary stewed fruit.

Take large winter pears, put them into a good hot oven, and keep turning them, so that they may not burn, for half an hour. Then peel them. Make a syrup of sugar and water — half a pound of sugar to quarter pint of water — put in the peeled pears, boil fast for five minutes, and then cover the pan and draw it aside to simmer till the fruit is quite soft.

You must take great care that the pears do not scorch while they are in the oven, or the scorched places will come up as dark marks on the finished fruit.

If you find it hard to peel the pears after roasting them, plunge each into cold water just for a moment before starting on them. But do not leave them to soak, or their flavor will be lost.

POIRES BONS CHRÉTIENS (GOOD CHRISTIAN PEARS).

"Why are they called that, Colette?"

"Because it is their name, the name both of the fruit and of the way of cooking it."

"Then, if one were to take other pears — Jargonelles, for instance — and cook them that way, would they be converted and become Good Christians?"

"Of course they would — at least they would be *Cooked* Good Christians — and so —. What are you laughing at *now*?"

Drop the peeled pears into a large pan of plain water and boil them till they begin to feel a little tender. Drain them well. Make a syrup of sugar and water just enough to cover them and add to it the juice and the thinly peeled rind of a lemon for each pound of sugar. Cover the pan and stew gently till the fruit is quite cooked. Put the pears standing up, as I told you before, in a rather large glass dish, strain the syrup around them, and put thin slices of lemon to float in the syrup. Serve very cold, iced if possible.

FRUIT TARTS of all kinds are exactly the same in France as all the world over, and so it is not worth my while to say much about them. Their only distinguishing feature is that the fruit is nearly always cooked in the pastry, with a large quantity of sugar, which, mingling with the juice, turns to a stiff syrup when the tart is cold.

Peel apples, slice them very thin, and arrange the slices in circles, overlapping each other. Sprinkle very thickly with sugar and let the tart brown so much that the sugar comes almost to the verge of burning.

Stone plums or cherries, and arrange them, as far as you can, in lines radiating out from the center.

Use a little red currant jelly with strawberries. They cook to such an ugly color if they are alone.

Cut apricots in half, stone them, and lay them with the cut side downwards. Colette says it is an open question as to whether you should peel them or not. They are much nicer when peeled; but, on the other hand, there is always danger that they will cook to a mash.

Don't make a tart of currants, unless they are black ones. A little red currant juice with cherries or raspberries is delicious, but the fruit alone is too full of seeds to be a nice tart.

Don't make a tart of pears either; it is very hard to manage, and not satisfactory, as the taste of the fruit is so

Colette Cooks Fruit

delicate that it is completely hidden by the taste of the pastry, and the result is *fade* in the extreme.

BEIGNETS, or fritters, are made of all kinds of unexpected things, over here. (You will find recipes for the fritter paste, and directions as to method, in the chapter on Frying.) But I think I might tell you here some of the fillings that Colette uses.

CHERRIES. Take those that are ripe enough to have the stone squeezed out. Thread five or six at a time on a fine skewer and dip them first in the fritter paste and then in the boiling fat. Shake them off into sifted sugar.

STRAWBERRIES AND RASPBERRIES. Throw them right into the fritter paste. Take them up on a drainer. Let the drainer drip a moment or two and then flick the fruits off it, one by one, with a skewer, into the hot fat. Take them out with another drainer and roll them in sifted sugar. Ever so good!

ROSE LEAVES. Use a rather thick fritter paste and the larger petals only of well-blown roses. Beat them quickly into the paste, and then take up a small teaspoonful at a time, and drop it into the hot fat. It puffs up and swims almost at once. Fish it out as soon as it is lightly browned, and you will find that the petals still keep their natural color. Drain the Beignets for a few seconds on kitchen paper, before rolling them in sifted sugar.

VINE LEAVES. Young and tender vine leaves are delicious, and so pretty. Choose those which are just well opened and leave each its stalk. Hold the leaf by the stalk, dip it in the fritter paste, give it a gentle little shake, and then dip it in the boiling fat. Never let go of the stalk at all till the fritter is quite cooked. When all are done, pile them high on a dish, and sprinkle them with sugar.

Colette's Best Recipes

ACACIA FLOWERS. Choose pretty bunches, of which the flowers are in full blow. Do them just like the vine leaves. They are absolutely charming, and very fragrant, as well as good.

It is best to fry all flowers and leaves in oil or butter; dripping might spoil their flavor a little.

ORANGES. Peel them carefully and separate them into sections. Rub the sections thickly with powdered sugar and leave them to soak for half an hour before dipping them in batter. Sugar them again after frying.

DRIED PLUMS, PRUNES, OR DATES. Soak dried plums or prunes in cold tea overnight. In all cases, replace the stone by a blanched almond. All three make delicious fritters.

CERISES PERLÉES (SUGARED CHERRIES) is a dessert that needs great delicacy of touch in the making; but it is worth the trouble, for it is extremely pretty and attractive, and it costs next to nothing.

Take large ripe cherries of the bright red sort; peel them delicately, cut their stalks to half the original length: roll them in fine sugar, making them pick up as much as they can. Spread them out on dishes, and put them in the full sun for one hour (in a glasshouse they will do better still). Then put them on ice, or in a very cold cellar, till the time of service comes. Stand them in a glass dish, with all their stems sticking up in the air, and surround them with whipped cream.

Red or white currants may be treated in the same way. But, as they naturally cannot be peeled, it is necessary to dip them in a little syrup and make them sticky, so that the sugar may cling to them. The fruit is held by the stalk when it is eaten. Both these sweets are very highly thought of in France and are served at what Colette calls "real dinners."

Colette Cooks Fruit

COMPOTE OF UNCOOKED CURRANTS is a very, very old recipe, and the dessert has a curiously delicate flavor which quite distinguishes it from modern cookery.

String half a pound of very ripe red currants. Wash and drain them. Add quarter pound of fine sugar and two tablespoonfuls of cold water. Toss all together till the sugar is perfectly melted, but do not stir in the least. Pour the whole into a glass dish and set it in a very cold cellar for two hours.

At the end of that time, you will find the currants set into a clear, soft red jelly, formed by their own juice and the sugar. If it is not set, put the dish on ice for a few minutes; but a too long icing is apt to set the jelly too stiff and rob it of some of the delicacy of texture, which is its great charm.

Hand with it a twin glass dish of Sweet Cheese (see page 187).

FRAISES À LA CHANTILLY (STRAWBERRIES À LA CHANTILLY) is a garden party, or summer dinner-party dish, just as good as it is pretty. Allow one pint of thick cream to one and a quarter pounds of strawberries. Pick out quarter pound of the finest and ripest of the berries. Wash the rest, and beat them through a sieve and sugar them. Whip the cream very stiff, mix the purée into it, pile all in a glass dish, and decorate with the berries that you have saved.

Raspberries can be treated in the same way. So, I should think, could blackberries, but I have never seen them, because we don't eat them much in France; they are thought good only for children to play with on the way to school!

COMPOTE D'ORANGES (COMPOTE OF ORANGES). Colette always says that oranges are no good for eating raw before March, — too sour. But she gives me a great many of them cooked, as we both agree that they are just as wholesome as they are nice.

Peel four oranges, divide them into sections, and take out the pips. The best way to do this is to make quite a small slit in the skin of the inner side, and work the pips up gently with your fingers. Boil together half a pound of sugar and quarter of a pint of water. When they have boiled for five minutes, pour them on the pieces of orange, which you have put into a china dish or bowl. Cover them and leave them for two hours.

Drain out the pieces of orange and pile them up high in a glass dish. Strain the syrup, boil it fast for five minutes more. Let it cool a little and then trickle it over the fruit. When all is quite cold, add piles of whipped cream here and there and serve.

ORANGES EN SURPRISE (SURPRISE ORANGES). Take large, ripe oranges. Cut off the top of one, just as you cut the top off a boiled egg. Take a tiny silver egg spoon and work it round and round gently inside the fruit, loosening the pulp from the skin and pounding it up. In a few minutes you will have room to add a little sugar. Keep on working with the spoon and adding sugar, and, if you like, a few grains of crushed ice, till all the inside of the fruit is reduced to pulp.

Stand the oranges up in a dish, surround them with crushed ice, and give a silver teaspoon with which to eat each.

PÊCHES AU BEURRE (BUTTERED PEACHES) are made exactly like Pommes au Beurre, and are very good indeed.

PÊCHES À LA CONDÉ (PEACHES A LA CONDÉ) is ever so pretty, and more of a real pudding than one generally gets in France.

Prepare quarter of a pound of rice, just as you did for

Colette Cooks Fruit

Pommes au Riz. While it is cooking, take ten fine peaches, dip them into boiling water, skin them, cut them in halves, and take out the stones. Stew them gently in a syrup made of quarter of a pound of sugar, four tablespoonfuls of water, and a few drops of vanilla, till they are quite soft.

Beat into your hot rice a tablespoonful of salt butter and the yolks of four eggs. Make a large round bed of the rice on a dish, arrange the halves of peaches on it, with a glacé cherry in the stonehole of each.

Take a pound pot of apricot jam, beat it up with enough of the peach syrup to make it just liquid, and pour it around and over the rice. It must not cover the peaches. Blanch two ounces of almonds, cut them into thin strips, and stick the jam thickly with them. Serve all warm.

The peaches have to be piled up a little on the rice, as there is not room for all to lie flat. But try to arrange things so that all the cherries show, as the little red dots peeping out from the fruit are very effective indeed.

Soufflé aux Abricots (Apricot Soufflé)
¼ pound butter
¼ pound sugar
3 ounces cornstarch
4 eggs
9 tablespoonfuls of the pulp of ripe apricots
Small sponge cakes

Beat the butter and sugar with a wooden spoon till the mixture becomes perfectly white. Then add the yolks of the eggs, one at a time, working each well in; the cornstarch; and the fruit pulp. Beat the whites of the eggs to the stiffest possible froth and stir them in.

Butter a plain three-pound cake tin and line the bottom and sides with sponge fingers, split open. Put in a good spreading of the apricot mixture; then more biscuits;

then more fruit. Do not fill the mold more than three quarters full. Set it in a large pan of water and let the water boil around it for half an hour. Then turn it out carefully on a hot dish. Beat up a pound pot of apricot jam with one fourth of its own bulk of boiling water. Put the mixture through a fine sieve over the soufflé.

"Do they know," asks Colette, "that, when I state a time for the cooking of something in the *bain-marie*, I mean that the time must be counted from the moment *when the water starts to boil?*"

"I'll tell. Is there anything else you want them to know?"

If you want to do good fruit cooking *always*

1. Do as much peeling and cutting as possible with a silver knife. A steel one is always likely to damage the color, even if it does not spoil the taste.

2. As you peel pears and apples, throw the pieces into water which contains a little vinegar. This will keep them a good color.

3. Never try to "get ahead" by peeling fruit hours before it is wanted. Even when kept in vinegar and water, it looses both texture and taste if left for more than half an hour or so.

4. Remember that fruit which is just *under*-ripe takes less sugar than that which is dead ripe.

5. A wee grain of salt added to fruit makes the sugar go much farther; but I have not mentioned this in the recipes, because it is one of the things that Colette *won't* take to. She calls it "new-fangled nonsense" and peacefully continues to waste the sugar.

CHAPTER XV

COLETTE MAKES CREAMS AND SWEET DISHES

SHE does not make many now — in fact, I never see one except on those rare occasions when friends come to luncheon or dinner — for a good French housekeeper would consider it almost a sin to serve creams to "the family" alone. A dish of fruit and a little cheese are quite enough, thank you! But, when we were all at home, and there very often used to be "real dinners", she attained to a pitch of excellence in cream and sweets-making, rarely arrived at by even a professional pastry cook.

If I give you a few of her recipes, will you please remember, in reading them, that the flavors suggested are not by any means the only ones that can be used. In your place, I should work out the book recipe exactly, just once, in order to make sure how it goes, and then vary the flavors, colors, shapes, etc., according to time of year and the tastes of your folks. In this way, you will get practically endless range of sweets, — all dainty and pretty, and none of them, I think, very hard to make.

Over here it is very usual to hand a little silver basket of Biscuits à la Cuiller with creams of any sort, especially with the very rich ones, which would hardly be nice alone.

You will notice the large extent to which eggs take the place of milk-cream. This is due to the fact that we are a cheese-making country, and milk-cream is, in consequence, rather rare and costly. But, if it is cheaper in America, you can often cut down the quantity of eggs by half and substitute cream for milk, with advantage to the dish.

CRÈME À LA VANILLE (VANILLA CREAM). To make ten little pots, take

> 1 quart rich milk
> 20 drops vanilla
> 3 ounces sugar
> The yolks of 3 eggs, and the white of 1

Warm the milk enough to make the sugar melt in it. Then let it get cold. Add the vanilla to it. Beat up the eggs as if for an omelette and pour in the milk, a little at a time, stirring all the while. Fill little pots and stand in the *bain-marie* till the cream "takes." Serve hot or cold in the pots. You may put a little jam or whipped cream on each, but this is *not* French; it is an English improvement.

The *bain-marie* means a saucepan — as flat and shallow as possible — on the bottom of which all the pots can stand. Pour in enough water to come rather more than halfway up them, and put the big pan on the fire to boil. There is no need to watch it, except just enough to see that the water is not boiling over into the creams. You must leave it open, — no cover at all, please. If you were to put a cover on, the steam would collect inside the cover, turn into water, and fall back into the creams, making them all watery and nasty.

You can tell pretty much by the look of the creams how they are getting on. When they look done, poke each right at the center with a straw. If liquid comes out, they are not yet cooked enough, but if the straw comes away dry, they are done.

Colette Makes Creams and Sweet Dishes

It's useless to poke the sides of them; sides get done in a very few minutes. Go right at the middle, please.

CRÈME RENVERSÉE (CARAMEL CREAM) is as much a standard dish in France as rice pudding in England, and far nicer.

Take a plain cake tin, which will hold rather more than a quart. Put into it eight lumps of sugar, pounded up and just dampened. Put your tin on the hottest part of the stove, so that the sugar browns quickly. When it is colored and melted, take hold of the mold — with the tongs, please, for it is horribly hot! — and turn it round and round, so that the sides may be coated as well as the bottom. Mind the sugar does not go too far and burn to blackness, won't you?

Make a crème just like the vanilla one, except that you add two extra eggs and use only half the amount of vanilla. Fill the prepared mold. Cook it just like the first creams. Serve it cold.

If you turn it out on the same day that it is made, you will find the tops and sides coated with brown. But if you leave it till next day, the caramel will liquefy and come streaming out all around the cream, like a sauce.

"Why does it do that, Colette?"

"Because that's its nature."

"And which is the nicer of the two, do you think?"

"It's a matter of taste."

So now you know as much about it as I do, — and that's not much!

CRÈME AU CHOCOLAT (CHOCOLATE CREAM). Grate three bars of good chocolate and melt them in a little of the milk. Then go on exactly as for Crème à la Vanille. Serve cold, with a generous dab of whipped cream on each pot.

Perhaps I had better just mention that Crème au Chocolat is one of those things to which can be applied the very wise saying that

> "There are nine and thirty ways
> Of inventing tribal lays.
> And every single one of them is right."

But Colette holds that the one I have just given you is the rightest.

CRÈME AU CAFÉ (COFFEE CREAM) is made exactly like Crème à la Vanille, except that you must use a little extra sugar, and have two tablespoonfuls of coffee essence instead of the vanilla.

If you want to make any of these crèmes in a big mold, and turn it out, use one extra egg — or, better still, two — to make it very firm. Don't put the whites in. Keep them back for other sweets, as they make the creams stringy, and do them no good.

That's an end of the plain crèmes. Now let us go on to a few fancy things.

BAVAROISE AU CAFÉ (COFFEE BAVAROISE). This is enough for two good-sized molds.

- 1 pint thick cream
- 1 pint fresh milk
- 4 sheets of white leaf gelatine
- 20 lumps sugar
- 6 eggs
- 2 tablespoonfuls coffee essence

Beat the eggs — yolks and whites together — for ten minutes. Warm the milk. Melt in it the sugar and gelatine. Add the coffee. Pour it slowly on the eggs, stirring all the while. Put the whole into a double pan and stir over the fire till the cream thickens. (You can do it in a single pan, if you like, but Colette says *she* wouldn't risk it herself, because a thing of this sort scorches in a second and is then perfectly uneatable. However, in an aluminum pan perhaps it might be all right.)

Let it cool down till you can put your finger into it without feeling anything special. Beat up the milk-cream till it is perfectly thick and then mix it well into the egg-cream. Pour both into wetted molds, and set them in a cold cellar all night.

Bavaroise may be eaten as soon as it is set — and that will be within a few minutes — if you put it on ice. But Colette thinks that it mellows and improves by being kept till next day.

It may be flavored with any kind of fruit syrup that you like, in place of the coffee, colored to match, and decorated with the fresh fruits.

BOMBE MARÉCHALE is quite simple, and what I call rather puddingy; but, for some reason or other, it is very highly thought of in France, and you will meet it on quite smart dinner tables, — beautifully decorated with whipped cream and glacé fruits, but Bomb Maréchale for all that.

Take a plain basin or cake tin and line the bottom and sides with Biscuits à la Cuiller, soaked in either sherry or fruit syrup. Make a Crème à la Vanille and add to it three sheets of gelatine, melted in a little of the milk, and fill the basin with it. Cook it in the *bain-marie*, with a plate over the basin or tin, and a weight on the plate, to keep the biscuits from swimming out of place. Turn it out when it is cold and decorate it to any extent you please.

BÛCHE AU CHOCOLAT. (Colette keeps, with great respect, an ancient tongue tin, in which she always makes Bûche, — one of those tall tongue tins, you know, that looks like a bit of drain pipe. I once asked her why she kept that horror, when she has a whole row of beautiful copper molds, twinkling unused on the top shelf, and she replied with dignity that a Bûche would not be a Bûche if it was n't made in a tongue tin. Nonsense, *I* call it. But you can do as you like about it.)

Dip your mold, whatever it may be, into milk. Grate five large bars of chocolate (weight about three quarters pound), and melt them in the smallest possible amount of boiling water. Let the chocolate get so cold that it is on the verge of setting. Then add the yolks of six eggs and mix very well. Beat the whites to a very stiff froth; add four tablespoonfuls of sugar to them.

Melt half an ounce of gelatine in a very little hot water and stir it into the chocolate. Fold in the whites of the eggs, lightly and gently, but mind they are well mixed; there must be no stripes or dabs. Pour all into your prepared tin and set aside in a cold place for six hours.

Turn it out on a dish and surround it with whipped cream. Sprinkle the whipped cream with a little grated chocolate.

This is very rich and needs to have biscuits handed with it.

DÉLICIEUX LYONNAIS is the prettiest thing you can think of, when it is made with all sorts of different-colored preserved fruits.

Beat the whites of six eggs to a very stiff froth and mix gently into them three tablespoonfuls of powdered sugar and four of preserved fruits, all kinds mixed, chopped into smallish pieces.

Butter very lightly one of those molds which have a hole in the middle, and put the mixture into it, leaving a little room for swelling. Cook it in the *bain-marie* till a straw thrust into it comes out clean. Turn it out into a

Colette Makes Creams and Sweet Dishes

glass dish and fill the hole at the center with Crème à la Vanille, made with the yolks of the eggs.

When Crème à la Vanille is wanted for such a purpose as this, it must not be cooked in pots; it must be stirred in a double pan over the fire till it thickens.

FROMAGE À LA CRÈME (SWEET CHEESE). This is a very delicious thing, which is served either alone or with fresh or stewed fruit. Many people like it better than whipped cow-cream with their fruit, because they find it less heavy and greasy.

Let a quart of milk go sour. If you want to hurry it up, put just a spot of vinegar into it and stand it near the fire. It must be so sour that it divides itself into solid and liquid parts.

Pour it into a clean cloth, hang the cloth up over a basin in the cellar, and leave it to drip all night. By next morning, the part in the cloth will be dry enough for use.

Put it into a basin, add rather less than half its own bulk of the finest possible sugar, and rub both together with a wooden spoon till they are perfectly smooth, — no little grains of sugar to be felt at all. Some people like a drop of vanilla flavoring, but I think, myself, that it is not wanted as the cheese has a definite taste of its own.

Add rich milk or thin cream, very gradually, stirring well all the time, till the mixture is the consistency of a custard or a mayonnaise sauce. Serve it in a glass dish.

The liquid part of the cheese is never used in France. But if you do any English cooking at all — boiled puddings or scones or anything of that kind — mix them with the liquid in place of milk or water; add a little bicarbonate of soda, and they will come up as light as feathers.

GÂTEAU MEXICAIN (MEXICAN CAKE). This is not a cake at all; it is a sort of frothy chocolate arrangement,

Colette's Best Recipes

which is handy for a party, because it must be made the day before.

4 eggs
Their weight in grated chocolate and in sifted sugar and in butter
Half their weight in flour

Melt the chocolate in a very little water and leave it on one side to get cool. Melt the butter. Stir in the sugar and flour. Beat in the yolks of the eggs, one at a time. Add the cooled chocolate. Last of all, whip the whites to the stiffest possible froth and fold it in. Put all into a couple of medium sized, buttered molds and cook in the *bain-marie* for one hour. Turn them out while they are still warm. Put them in glass dishes when they are cold and surround them with whipped cream or a custard.

It is rather pretty to use two or three tins, each smaller than the other, and to build up the cold chocolate shapes into a tower, sticking them together by a spreading of whipped cream.

ÎLE FLOTTANTE (FLOATING ISLAND). Beat the whites of four eggs to the stiffest possible froth; fold into them a couple of tablespoonfuls of powdered sugar. Put all into a carameled tin (see Crème Renversée), and cook in the *bain-marie* till a straw which is thrust into the fluff comes out clean.

Meanwhile, make a Crème à la Vanille with the yolks. Cook it in a pan — not in pots — and don't let it get too thick. Allow it to cool.

Turn out the white mass into a large glass dish or bowl and trickle the custard around it. It will stand up and float.

ŒUFS À LA NEIGE (SNOW EGGS), that most celebrated of French sweets, is made just the same, except that, instead of being all cooked together in a mold, the whipped whites are taken up, a spoonful at a time, and just poached

Colette Makes Creams and Sweet Dishes

in a pan of boiling water. When you remove them from the water, let them drain for a few minutes on a plate, as they give off a good deal of liquid, which would make the Crème thin and poor if they were put straight into it.

LE RÊVE (THE DREAM) is practically the same thing as Île Flottante, except that you must stir half a pound of crystallized rose leaves into your whites before cooking them. A drop of carmine in the Crème adds greatly to the prettiness of the whole affair.

MOUSSE. See "Mousse aux Pommes" in chapter on Fruit Cookery. A Mousse may be very well made with chocolate, melted in a very few drops of hot water: or with fruit pulp of any kind, provided that there is not too much juice in it. It is a very economical plan to make a Mousse and a Crème together, using the yolks of the eggs for one and the whites for another.

SOUFFLÉ DE MARRONS (CHESTNUT SOUFFLÉ). Boil twenty-five large chestnuts in plain water till they are soft. Carefully take away all the skin, and put the nuts through a sieve. Add to them the yolks of four eggs, well beaten, and quarter pound of sifted sugar. Mix very well and then add a piece of fresh butter the size of an egg, the juice of a lemon, and, last, the whites of the eggs beaten to a very stiff froth. Butter a round soufflé dish, put in the mixture — which should not fill it more than about half — and cook it fifteen minutes in a very hot oven. Serve at once.

If you like to leave it till it is quite cold and then serve it with whipped cream, it will be good also, though of a different texture, — close and smooth, instead of being all light and fluffy.

Many people prefer orange juice to lemon. Try both and choose for yourself.

SAMBAYONNES. For each person allow one egg, one

Colette's Best Recipes

tablespoonful sifted sugar, one tablespoonful Madeira wine, or, if you don't use wine, orange juice.

Separate the yolks from the whites. Beat the yolks with the sugar till the mixture becomes quite white. Add the flavoring. Whip the whites of the eggs to a stiff froth and fold them in gently. Pile up the mixture in champagne glasses, sprinkle the surface with glacé fruits chopped small, and offer a teaspoon with each glass.

Whenever possible, pack the glasses in chopped ice, but do not mix any ice into the cream, or you will make it taste thin and poor.

PALAIS DE GLACE (CRYSTAL PALACE). Put three ounces of sugar into a small pan and burn it a good brown. (Take care it does not go black.) When it is nicely colored, add two tablespoonfuls of boiling water and stir hard, till the whole affair makes a caramel syrup.

In a large basin, melt half an ounce of gelatine in half a gill of boiling water. Beat the whites of six eggs to the stiffest possible froth, fold them into the melted gelatine, and add the caramel, and also, if you like, a very little powdered sugar. Mix thoroughly, but gently. Pour all into a mold which has been dipped in cold water and set it in a cold place for six hours at least. Turn out and surround with a thick, well-sweetened custard.

"Perhaps, Colette, we had better give them a few recipes for real *entremets* — things made with rice, and so on."

"Well, all those creams are *entremets;* what better do you want?"

"I don't want anything better. I want something rather less good, something plainer and more satisfying, you know."

RIZ À L'IMPÉRATRICE (EMPRESS RICE). Wash five tablespoonfuls of rice and boil it in five wine-glassfuls of milk.

Colette Makes Creams and Sweet Dishes

At the end of half an hour, add twelve lumps of sugar. Let the rice boil gently till it is quite soft and thick.

I hope it won't burn; it won't in all probability, if you keep it right at the side of the stove. But, still, scorched rice is a trouble that one does meet, now and again, in kitchens. If it should happen to you, stand the pan right away in cold water — to cool it down and keep the burnt fumes from rising — and take off the rice from the top, lightly, with a spoon, smelling each spoonful. As soon as you come to one that smells burnt, don't take any more; the rest is only good for the chickens. By this means, you can often save half or three quarters of the panful: but if you stir it up recklessly, and then scrape out the burnt part along with the good, none of it will be eatable at all.

Let the rice cool. When you can hold your finger in it easily, beat one pint of cream quite stiff and stir it in. Add five sheets of gelatine, melted in a few drops of hot water, and any flavoring that you like best. Put all into a large, wetted mold, and stand in a cold place or on ice. Turn out and surround with red currant or raspberry jelly.

The amount of cream may be reduced if you want to be economical.

SOUFFLÉ DE RIZ (RICE SOUFFLÉ). Cook five tablespoonfuls of rice, as above. When it has cooled a little, beat into it one tablespoonful of melted butter, a small pinch of salt, sugar and the yolks of two or three eggs. Whip up the whites to a very stiff froth and fold them in gently. Fill a buttered soufflé dish not more than half full and put it into a brisk oven for twenty minutes.

The rice should rise very much. It should have a nice golden crust, which generally breaks into a peak at the middle, and lets the lighter inside boil out a little, just like a very perfectly baked cake.

Colette's Best Recipes

Serve very hot. No sauce or fruit is wanted with it.

If you want to make good creams and sweets, always

1. Remember that they are very delicate things, which spoil quickly and must not be kept hanging round in the hot kitchen for even a needless second. When you take them out to the cellar or the cold larder, remember that you should not stand them near meat or soup or anything strong-scented, as they have a wonderful readiness to suck up scents and tastes which do not belong to them, especially when they are still hot. For this reason, you never ought to make creams in molds that have ever been used for meat or fish. They may be quite clean — they may have been boiled out dozens of times — but, all the same, you can never be sure that a certain greasiness does not cling to them, and that, if it does not actually "tang" your cream, it may spoil its first freshness.

2. Don't touch and fuss creams too much. The less handling they get, the better they will be.

3. If you think they are going to be troublesome to turn out, dip the mold quickly in and out of a bowl of boiling water, and then the contents will simply skate out into the dish. But don't let the mold remain in the hot water for more than a bare second, or the cream will be so much melted that the outlines of it will be blurred and spoiled.